BEGINNER'S GUIDE TO
REFLECTIVE PRACTICE IN NURSING

Sara Miller McCune founded SAGE Publishing in 1965 to support the dissemination of usable knowledge and educate a global community. SAGE publishes more than 1000 journals and over 800 new books each year, spanning a wide range of subject areas. Our growing selection of library products includes archives, data, case studies and video. SAGE remains majority owned by our founder and after her lifetime will become owned by a charitable trust that secures the company's continued independence.

Los Angeles | London | New Delhi | Singapore | Washington DC | Melbourne

BEGINNER'S GUIDE TO
REFLECTIVE PRACTICE IN NURSING
CATHERINE DELVES-YATES

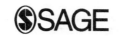SAGE

Los Angeles | London | New Delhi
Singapore | Washington DC | Melbourne

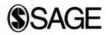

Los Angeles | London | New Delhi
Singapore | Washington DC | Melbourne

SAGE Publications Ltd
1 Oliver's Yard
55 City Road
London EC1Y 1SP

SAGE Publications Inc.
2455 Teller Road
Thousand Oaks, California 91320

SAGE Publications India Pvt Ltd
B 1/I 1 Mohan Cooperative Industrial Area
Mathura Road
New Delhi 110 044

SAGE Publications Asia-Pacific Pte Ltd
3 Church Street
#10-04 Samsung Hub
Singapore 049483

Editor: Alex Clabburn
Assistant Editor: Ozlem Merakli
Development editor: Eleanor Rivers
Senior project editor: Chris Marke
Marketing manager: George Kimble
Cover design: Sheila Tong
Typeset by: C&M Digitals (P) Ltd, Chennai, India
Printed in the UK

Library of Congress Control Number: 2020945555

British Library Cataloguing in Publication data

A catalogue record for this book is available from
the British Library

ISBN 978-1-4739-6920-9
ISBN 978-1-4739-6921-6 (pbk)

At SAGE we take sustainability seriously. Most of our products are printed in the UK using responsibly sourced
papers and boards. When we print overseas we ensure sustainable papers are used as measured by the PREPS
grading system. We undertake an annual audit to monitor our sustainability.

CONTENTS

LIST OF FIGURES

LIST OF TABLES

ABOUT THE AUTHOR

Catherine Delves-Yates is an experienced nurse and a lecturer at the School of Health Sciences, University of East Anglia, UK. She started her nursing career at the Nightingale School of Nursing, London, and has worked clinically in adult and paediatric critical care in the UK, and has nursed and taught in America, Africa and Nepal. Her passion is to ensure that all nurses have the knowledge, skills and professionalism to deliver effective compassionate care to each of their patients. Catherine is an Honorary Lecturer at the University of Buea and the Higher Institute of Applied Medical Sciences, Cameroon, and an international adviser to the Patan Academy of Health Sciences, Nepal. Currently, she is researching whether nursing students' views of health and illness alter during their pre-registration nursing programme.

ABOUT THE CONTRIBUTORS

Coral Drane graduated from the University of East Anglia (UEA) as a Registered Nurse in 2014, having changed careers after 20 years teaching in Further Education. She is an NMC Registered Nurse Teacher and a Fellow of the Higher Education Institute. She began her nursing career at the Norfolk and Norwich University Hospital (NNUH) within Cardiology. In 2015, Coral reconnected with teaching, becoming an Associate Tutor, then an Adult Nurse Lecturer at UEA, while continuing part-time nursing. In January 2020, Coral decided to focus on her clinical role in Cardiology, while remaining an Associate Tutor at UEA. In December 2020, she was seconded as a Practice Development Nurse at NNUH. She is passionate about education, Cardiology and interprofessional learning, and recognises the vital importance of reflection in developing clinical practice.

Gail Selby is a newly qualified nurse working within the specialism of Endoscopy at the Norfolk and Norwich University Hospital. She has worked within the Endoscopy unit for eleven and a half years as a Health Care Assistant and more recently as an Assistant Practitioner, before completing the Nurse Degree Apprenticeship Programme. Gail undertook her nurse training as a mature student and relishes the additional responsibility that being a registered nurse brings, as well as developing her skills and knowledge within her field. Gail feels strongly that patients should have a positive experience when attending the hospital and is a staunch advocate of this. She achieved a First Class Honours Degree.

Rebekah Hill is an Associate Professor within the School of Health Sciences, University of East Anglia. Her role involves teaching and assessing both undergraduate and postgraduate health-care practitioners across a range of professions. As the Director of Education for the school, she has a special interest in assessment of learning. Rebekah works clinically as an Advanced Life Support Instructor and within gastroenterology nursing, maintaining her special interest in hepatitis C.

AUTHOR'S ACKNOWLEDGEMENTS

Thank you to:

All the patients, nurses and nursing students who have provided me with the experience and experiences needed to write this book.

Coral Drane for all her hard work and Rebekah Hill for her ideas.

Gail Selby for being such an excellent student and outstanding nurse.

All at SAGE, especially Ozlem Merakli, who provided inspiration when I had none.

And finally, Martin and Florence Delves-Yates for their support, encouragement and playing balleee.

PUBLISHER'S ACKNOWLEDGEMENTS

The author and publisher are grateful to the following academics for their work reviewing the proposal and draft material of this text:

Ellen Kitson-Reynolds, University of Southampton.

Rosie Stenhouse, University of Edinburgh.

Peter Ellis, Independent Nursing Educational Consultant and Writer.

INTRODUCTION

This book has been written for registered nurses and nursing students alike, no matter what field of nursing you are working in, intend to work in, how long you have been registered or how far through your nursing programme you are. The book presents a solid foundation of relevant material to build your reflective practice skills upon, and is designed to support you through your journey from a beginner 'doing reflection' to a practitioner who understands the importance of 'being reflective'.

No matter how long we have been using reflection in our nursing practice, we are all at different stages on our reflective practice journey. At times this can be daunting, exciting, frustrating and empowering, or maybe even all of these at the same time. This book has been written as a guide to motivate you to keep going and to encourage you to celebrate excellence in your nursing care.

BOOK STRUCTURE

The book is designed to present you with an understandable and applicable approach to reflective practice. This is done in a range of ways.

The material considered has been split into the following themes, each of which forms a part of the book:

Part A – Understanding Reflection

Part B – Applying Reflection

Part C – Going Further

Each of these parts is further divided into chapters, supporting you to develop both your reflective practice knowledge and skill, and then integrate it into your nursing practice. Each part of the book starts with a case study and reflection, which is reviewed and further developed in the chapters within the part, providing a real-life approach to reflection.

To further aid your understanding, all chapters include activities which encourage you to engage with the material being considered and to apply it to your individual learning.

Further to this, each chapter starts with:

- voices from nursing students and registered nurses, outlining questions that will be considered;
- a clear identification of what will be covered.

Finally, each chapter ends with:

- a glossary, where there is an explanation of any words in the text that are in **bold** type;
- a recommended book, article and web-link, which will enable you to take your understanding further than the information presented within the chapter.

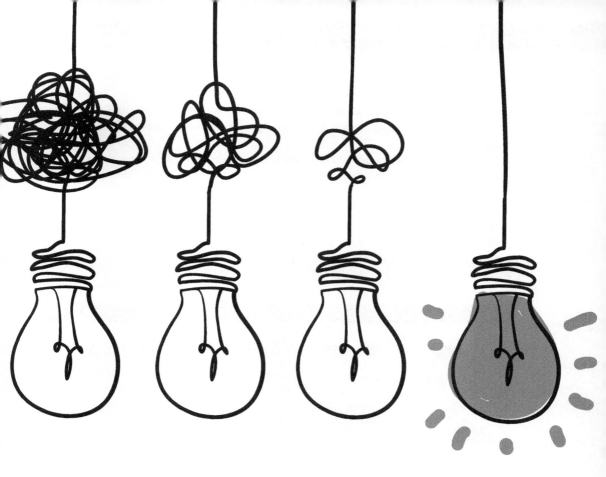

PART A

UNDERSTANDING REFLECTION

This first part of the textbook will enable you to understand the importance of reflection in nursing; how it can increase your self-awareness as well as enable you to improve your nursing practice. We will consider how you can write an effective reflection, how you can think and write critically, plus introduce a good model of reflection to use for your first reflections.

At the start of each chapter you will hear from a registered nurse and nursing student, who are likely to be sharing the challenges and asking the questions you are, as you start your journey towards 'being reflective'.

Before you read the chapters in this part, however, I would like to introduce you to Angus Plumb, who is going to share his thoughts and first reflection with you. As we progress through this part of the book, we will refer back to Angus's work and identify how it could be further developed.

CASE STUDY

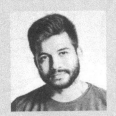

ANGUS PLUMB, FIRST YEAR NURSING STUDENT, MENTAL HEALTH FIELD

Angus is 19 years old and has wanted to be a nurse since he was admitted to hospital aged 7 to have his appendix removed.

After completing his A-levels, Angus took a year out to work as a volunteer teacher at a school in Kisumu, Kenya. He loved the time he spent at the school and enjoyed living away from home, in another country, with a different culture.

Angus is half-way through the first module of his nursing programme. Yesterday was his first day on placement, which he thoroughly enjoyed, although at times it was rather daunting. Angus has been asked by his **practice supervisor** to write an informal reflection focusing on his first day in placement.

HI! ANGUS HERE!

I had a really good first day on placement yesterday. It was jolly scary at times, though, and I didn't sleep at all the night before. One of the funniest things was putting on my uniform. I looked like a nurse, but didn't feel like one. Actually, when I was on the ward someone called out 'nurse' and I looked behind me to see where they were. Then I realised they were talking to me! I really can't believe that this is happening – I'm starting on my journey to become a nurse. I've wanted to do this for years, but now it is actually happening. Yippee!! Brilliant, brilliant, brilliant!!!

I'm excited, but worried too. On my course there are lots of students who have been **HCAs**. In the skills sessions they know exactly what to do. I don't. Yesterday, I felt really out of my depth. I think I managed to do everything OK, but that was more down to luck. I found it difficult to know what to do; everything is so very confusing.

The patients were really great. They helped me loads even when I was very slow. Luckily, nothing happened where I had to be quick and thank goodness there wasn't an emergency, as I kept forgetting where the sluice was, let alone remembering anything else. I want to be like my practice supervisor - she is soooooo good. She knows all of the patients by name and can remember what is wrong with them. I found that difficult too.

I'm getting annoyed with myself – when I was in Africa working in the school, I knew what I needed to do, so why am I being so slow now?

The nurses on the ward were really helpful and said they could remember their first day. They all said that if I wanted to know anything, I only just had to ask, which was great. Trouble is, though, that I know so little I don't realise what questions I should ask. I'm on placement with three other students from my group, so when things got too bad I was able to seek them out for support. They seemed to be getting on really well; it only seems to be me who is feeling overwhelmed.

I'm back on placement later today and my practice supervisor has asked me to write a reflection about my first day. She said doing this would help me realise what I had learnt and what I needed to learn. At the moment I feel that I need to learn everything, and quickly!!!! I'm going to use Borton's (1970) model for my reflection, as when we talked about reflection in class I thought this way of reflecting was the easiest to understand.

I feel that the topic I need to focus on is that there is so much to learn – way too much – and after thinking about it, I'm starting to worry that there is just no way I'm going to be able to do this.

ANGUS'S REFLECTION

WHAT?

Yesterday was the first day of my first clinical placement. I really enjoyed it, but I feel that there is so very much to learn and I am worried that I am never going to get the hang of it. I feel that everyone else knows so much more than me and I am finding it hard to be confident about my abilities.

SO WHAT?

If I don't know enough I might do the wrong thing. This could result in a patient not getting the right treatment. This does worry me, as we have had lots of sessions about the importance of The Code (NMC, 2018) and I want to give patients good care.

Thinking a bit more about this, and remembering how I felt on my first day when I was a volunteer teacher in the school in Africa, I realise that I felt the same! Until now, I had forgotten that it took me a couple of weeks to feel that I had any idea as to what I needed to do there.

NOW WHAT?

I need to make sure that I only do the things I know are correct and if I am not sure, I have got to ask and not feel that I am an annoyance to the other ward staff when I do this. My practice supervisor is there to guide me; she is great at this, so I need to work closely with her. I am going to try doing this to see if it stops me feeling so out of my depth.

I need to give myself time and not expect that I can go into a new situation, be an expert and feel comfortable straight away.

(Continued)

ANGUS'S THOUGHTS FOLLOWING HIS REFLECTION

When my practice supervisor suggested that I do a reflection about my first day, I really didn't think that I would gain anything from it – but I did! It was very helpful to take a bit of time and think about what had happened plus how I was feeling. I now realise that I was expecting far too much of myself and that I need to have more patience. I have wanted to be a nurse for such a long time and I was expecting to be as good as my practice supervisor, but this is silly as she has so much more experience than me.

I am now feeling more confident that I can do it! I am sure it will be hard work, but it will be worth it.

GLOSSARY

HCAs   Healthcare assistants. Members of nursing staff who help deliver care.

practice supervisor   A professional registered with the NMC, GMC or HCPC who supervises nursing students while they are in a practice learning environment.

REFERENCES

Borton, T. (1970) *Reach, Touch and Teach*. London: Hutchinson.
Nursing and Midwifery Council (NMC) (2018) *The Code*. London: NMC.

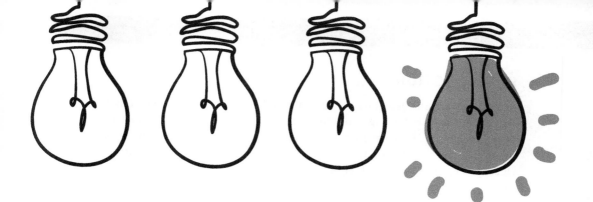

WHAT IS REFLECTION?

CATHERINE DELVES-YATES

1

> I'm starting to panic. My first assignment is due in two weeks – I have to do a reflection on my experience during my placement. I have been to the sessions on reflection, but I am still confused about what I need to do. What is a reflective model? What should I reflect on?
>
> I went to the library to find a book to help, but that used lots of words I don't understand and now I'm getting really worried . . .
>
> **Alex Charles, nursing student, child field**

> I'm not sure what I need to do for the reflections for my revalidation. I have lots of experiences I think will be good, but how should I write them down?
>
> **Larry Chi, registered nurse, learning disability field**

INTRODUCTION

Reflection is a term that is used in nursing to describe many different activities, which can make it both confusing and difficult to define. Reflection includes a wide range of practices spanning from the relatively simple 'doing reflection', which involves reflection on an experience to 'being reflective', which involves a constant state of mindfulness, where nurses are continually vigilant against unskilful actions and negative attitudes that could cloud their judgement (Johns, 2017).

In its simplest form, reflection can be described as a process we frequently undertake without really thinking about it. Think about the last time you treated yourself to something you thought was nice. How did you decide what 'nice' was? Probably by reflecting on your previous experience. Just imagine walking into a garden on a hot sunny day and absent-mindedly picking what you thought was a 'nice' ripe plum tomato, taking a bite out of it and realising that what you have just bitten into was not a ripe plum tomato but actually a very hot chilli. You would be reflecting on your mistaken choice of 'nice' not only as you ran to the closest source of a drink, but also while you drank enough to put out the fire inside you. The sort of reflection that Alex and Larry, who we heard from at the start of this chapter, need to undertake, shares many similarities with this 'tomato–chilli incident', particularly in that they are all likely to have the same result of changing future actions.

As Alex and Larry tell us, reflection is an important skill that nursing students and registered nurses need to understand. Many, if not all, universities use reflection to assess the development of a nursing student's knowledge and attitudes, and the **Nursing and Midwifery Council (NMC)** requires nurses registered in the United Kingdom to undertake reflection as a way to demonstrate that they are constantly learning and keeping up to date.

Taking a simple 'doing reflection' approach, this chapter will outline the fundamental role that reflection has in enabling you to learn from experience, to ensure that you can deliver the best care possible to patients. First, we will consider what reflection is, plus why there is a need for both nursing students and registered nurses to reflect, followed by how reflection can be used to help you learn. Finally, what is needed in order to produce a reflection will be discussed and a simple model that aids reflection will be introduced.

———————————— CHAPTER AIMS ————————————

This chapter will enable you to:

- understand what reflection means in nursing;
- recognise the reasons why nurses need to reflect;
- realise how reflection will be useful to you;
- make a good start when producing your own reflections.

WHAT IS REFLECTION IN NURSING?

Reflection is a term frequently used to describe learning from experience. While this is a reasonable starting point, a better definition of reflection is 'thinking with a purpose'.

If reflection is thought of in this way, it becomes easy to understand that reflection is an active and at times uncomfortable process, as you may need to consider difficult topics. Thinking in this way involves a number of different elements, so when you hear people talking about reflection, you are likely also to hear a number of other terms being used. Before considering any further what reflection is, it is necessary to understand what is meant by these other terms. To make this more complicated, not only do many of these terms sound similar, they are often used **interchangeably**. Knowing this is all part of the process of becoming a **reflective practitioner**, for once you have mastered these terms, you will also be able to join in any conversation about reflection and will sound like an expert.

As has been said, reflection is 'thinking with a purpose', with the purpose being learning from an experience. When considered in this way, the term 'reflection' highlights another term you will often hear, **reflective practice**, which is what has just been described: thinking about an experience and learning from it. Reflective practice is an important way to learn from experience, especially the experiences you have in a professional context. In order to help you to learn from your experience, **reflective processes** are applied. These are a range of specifically structured methods that will help you to think about an experience, learn from it and, most importantly, turn your learning into actions. When you function in this way, you are being a reflective practitioner, using what you have learnt from your experience to ensure that you develop your nursing knowledge and deliver the best care you possibly can.

In this chapter, we will consider some simple definitions to help you to gain a sound understanding of what reflection is. Table 1.1 provides a summary of these definitions. When considering reflection, you will hear or see the terms **reflective** and **reflexive** being used. These terms can both, very simply, be thought of as meaning 'being thoughtful' and are often used interchangeably. In more accurate terms, reflexive relates to exploring, examining and critiquing your claims or assumptions as the result of an encounter with another person, culture, idea or experience. In general, you will find that reflective is used more often than reflexive, although both the process of writing a reflection and the written reflection itself can be referred to as **reflexive writing**, whereas the process of talking with another person about a reflection and the spoken reflection itself can be referred to as a **reflective discussion**.

Reflexivity is the foundation of all these processes. While you may well find that when you are reflecting, you focus on experiences involving others, reflection is actually about you learning how you behave in different situations. Having insight into your behaviour is a very powerful tool, as this gives you the ability to change and enables your practice to be **mindful**.

Table 1.1 Getting to grips with some important terms

Term	Meaning
Reflection	Thinking with a purpose.
Reflective practitioner	A nurse (or other healthcare professional) who uses what they have learnt from experience to develop their knowledge and deliver the best care possible.
Reflective practice	Thinking about an experience and learning from it.

(Continued)

Table 1.1   (Continued)

Term	Meaning
Reflective processes	Specifically structured methods that enable new actions to be based on learning gained from experience.
Reflexive or reflective	In the simplest form, both are used to mean being purposefully thoughtful. Reflexive more accurately relates to deliberately looking back on your claims or assumptions, exploring, examining and critiquing them, usually following an encounter with another person, or a new culture, idea or experience.
Reflexive writing	The process of writing a reflection and the written reflection itself.
Reflective discussion	The process of talking with another person about a reflection and the spoken reflection itself.
Reflexivity	Using experiences to learn more about you.

As we have said, in this chapter we are taking a simple approach to reflection in order to enable you to gain a clear understanding of a number of important terms. This will ensure that you feel confident in your ability to become a reflective practitioner, unlike Alex and Larry at the start of this chapter.

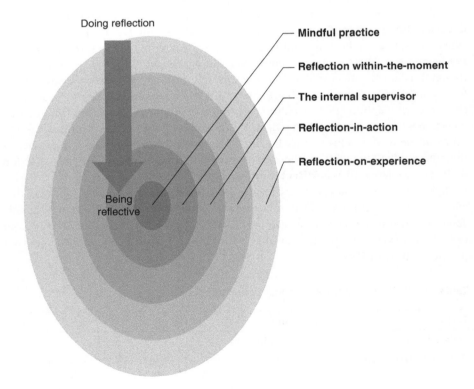

Figure 1.1   Reflection as an onion

Source: Adapted from Johns (2017) *Becoming a Reflective Practitioner* (5th edn). Hoboken, NJ: Wiley-Blackwell. Reproduced by kind permission of John Wiley & Sons.

One of the best ways to think of reflection is to imagine it as being like an onion. Reflection has many 'layers' which you need to peel away in order to get from the simple approach of 'doing reflection' to the more complex 'being reflective' at the core.

As shown in Figure 1.1, once you have got to grips with 'doing reflection', you need to work on peeling the layers of the onion away, so you can begin 'being reflective.'

ACTIVITY 1.1

Before reading any further, considering what you have read so far and any relevant experiences you may have had, if you were asked 'Why is there a need for nurses to reflect?', what would you say?

Check the activity answers at the end of the chapter to see if we agree.

WHY IS THERE A NEED FOR NURSES TO REFLECT?

It has been said for many years that reflection is beneficial to professional practice because:

1.　it enables nurses to learn from their experiences;
2.　it improves their confidence in both justifying the actions they take and supporting their decision making (Glaze, 2002).

Thus, reflection has the ability to empower nurses, because the knowledge it brings enables them to take control of their circumstances, become more assertive and problem solve imaginatively.

Reflection provides an aspect of **retrospective contemplation**, which is of great value because this has the potential to facilitate self-knowledge and self-development in the person who is reflecting. So, if a nursing student, like Angus in Part A, reflects on an experience, they can learn about themselves, and make plans to change or develop their actions, attitudes or knowledge.

Thus, the answer to the question 'Why do nurses need to reflect?' is to ensure that the care they deliver to patients is always the best possible. While being a reflective practitioner can bring the personal benefits of being able to learn from experience, being confident, assertive and knowing yourself, it is these qualities that will enable you to ensure that, in every situation, you are doing all you can, not only to uphold your professional code (NMC, 2018), but also to demonstrate the attributes of good nursing (DH, 2012), as identified in Figure 1.2.

Being a reflective practitioner is the key to achieving the expectation that all registered nurses must keep themselves up to date and apply the most recent and best evidence to their practice (NMC, 2018). In order to successfully complete their nursing programme, nursing students also need to abide by these standards. Expectations such as these are of the utmost importance, as they ensure that both patients and the public in general are able to have confidence in the care they receive.

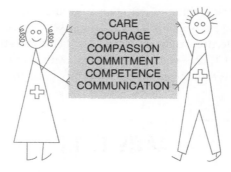

Figure 1.2   The attributes of good nursing

Source: Delves-Yates (2018) *Essentials of Nursing Practice* (2nd edn). London: Sage.

HOW WILL REFLECTION BE USEFUL TO YOU?

Some of the answers to the question 'How will reflection be useful to you?' really depends on who you are. If you are a nursing student, like Alex who we met at the start of this chapter, being able to produce a good written reflection will allow you to submit your assignment and get a high mark. If you are a registered nurse, like Larry who we also met at the start of the chapter, being able to present formal written reflections and undertake a reflective discussion will enable you to achieve **revalidation** with the NMC. These are, however, only partial answers to the question – a starting point. If you consider what we have said in the previous section highlighting why there is a need to reflect, it becomes clear that reflection has far more potential than just getting a high mark and revalidating.

THE BENEFITS OF REFLECTION

Reflection can be thought of as an important learning tool or a journey of learning (Johns, 2017). By purposely thinking about previous experience, it is possible to learn from them and apply this knowledge to actions in the future. Reflecting on experience allows you to recognise both your strengths and your limitations. As human beings, there is a tendency to focus on the things we are not good at, ignoring our strengths. As a professional practitioner, however, this is not a sound strategy. To uphold *The Code* (NMC, 2018) we need a clear understanding of all our skills, knowledge and attitudes. This includes both what we are good at, as well as what we need to improve. By thinking of reflection as a learning tool or a journey of learning, we can use it to become more effective in all areas of our skill, knowledge and attitudes. Such an approach makes us a reflective practitioner, which not only improves patient care, but also brings a sense of personal satisfaction.

ACTIVITY 1.2

Think with a purpose (or 'reflect') about an activity you were undertaking before starting to read this book. Set yourself a time limit of 5 minutes to write down:

what you did well;

what you would have liked to have done better.

There is no definitive answer to this activity as the question is based on your own reflection.

REFLECTING ON 'GOOD' OR 'BAD' EXPERIENCES

As has already been considered, it is always more tempting to reflect on experiences where things may not have gone as well as had been anticipated – for example, the tomato–chilli incident at the start of the chapter. The matter of 'good' or 'bad' experiences will be covered later in this section, but before doing this, it is necessary to consider what exactly 'experience' is, because to produce an effective reflection you need to have a clear understanding of this. Figure 1.3 highlights what can be meant when talking about experience.

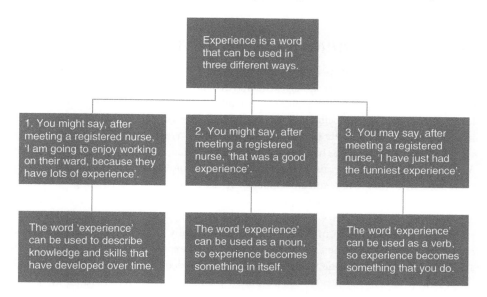

Figure 1.3   What can be meant when talking about 'experience'?

In addition to being able to use the word 'experience' in three different ways, experience can be of many different types – for example, **cognitive**, physical, emotional, spiritual, religious, virtual, social or subjective.

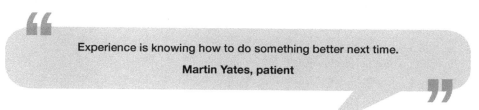

Experience is knowing how to do something better next time.

Martin Yates, patient

A further way to think of experience in nursing is, as Martin suggests, how you gain practical expertise. This differs from the theoretical knowledge you gain from books and lectures. Reflecting on what you do, how you do it and how you feel about it is an excellent way to link practical nursing with theoretical knowledge. We will discuss this topic in more detail in the chapters in Part B.

Having considered what is meant by the term 'experience' and relating this to nursing, it is now possible to return to the matter of whether reflection should focus on 'good' or 'bad' experiences. Thinking about labelling an experience as 'good' or 'bad', an expert reflective practitioner would tell you that 'Experience is constant and continuous, so it is neither good nor bad, it is just experience'.

They would then go on to say that the way to act when an experience is not going smoothly is to pause and consider the best way to continue. This is called reflection in action, which we will discuss in Part B of this book. However, as we are at the start of our learning journey to understand reflection, in this chapter we are taking a simpler 'doing reflection' approach. So, when we look back at an experience, it may either have ended in a way we felt happy about, or in a way that made us worried. Whichever it was doesn't actually matter, because it is possible to learn from both experiences.

ACTUALLY LEARNING FROM REFLECTION

Throughout your life so far, as a mechanism to ensure your survival, you will have developed a number of everyday learning strategies that have a reflective element. Think back to the case of mistaken identity between the tomato and chilli – this is an example of such an everyday learning strategy, which hopefully results in only mistaking a chilli for a tomato once in a lifetime! However, it isn't exactly how we reflect in nursing. When we are reflecting in nursing, we need to consider what has happened in much more detail, carefully analysing our actions, feelings and the outcome, considering what could be improved for the future. It is actually more accurate to think of the tomato–chilli experience as an example of learning by accident.

Reflection differs from learning by accident. Learning from reflection is a deliberate act, so it does not happen accidentally. When you reflect, you think purposefully about a situation, carefully considering the experience, specifically focusing on what you did and how you felt. It is often the case that reflecting on an experience enables you to understand what needs to be done to improve the care provided to patients, so reflections are often written down, not just for the purposes of assignments or revalidation, but as the first step in improving patient care.

ACTIVITY 1.3

Think with a purpose about every action you undertake when cleaning your teeth: think about what you do, how you do it and how you feel as you do it while:

1. finding your toothpaste;
2. lifting up your toothbrush;

3. putting toothpaste on your toothbrush;
4. lifting your toothbrush to your mouth;
5. moving the brush up and down;
6. spitting out the toothpaste;

etc., etc., etc., . . .

There is no definitive answer to this activity as the question is based on your own reflection.

If you applied the level of purposeful thinking used in Activity 1.3 to every aspect of your life it wouldn't be helpful, as you would be constantly questioning yourself and not accomplish anything. This means that while reflection is an excellent way to learn, it is best used for specific experiences.

PRESENTING YOUR REFLECTION

CASE STUDY 1.1: ANNABELLE AVRANCHES

Annabelle completed a nursing programme and became a registered nurse, adult field, 20 years ago. After working in A&E for three years, she left nursing to run her own garden design business. Annabelle recently decided that she wanted to work as a nurse again, so started a return-to-nursing course two weeks ago. Reflection wasn't something taught on her nursing programme 20 years ago or used in the three years that she worked in A&E.

Annabelle has been asked to produce a reflection focusing on the skills she can transfer to nursing from her experience of running a business. She has thought purposefully about her experience of running a business and has come up with a list of six skills.

When Annabelle shares what she has done with the other students in her class, she finds that she is the only one who has written a list; most of the others have written what seems to be more like an essay, although one other classmate has drawn a picture.

Annabelle is happy that the skills she has identified will be really useful and that devising her list helped her to learn from her experience. She is, however, very confused about how she should write her reflection.

(Continued)

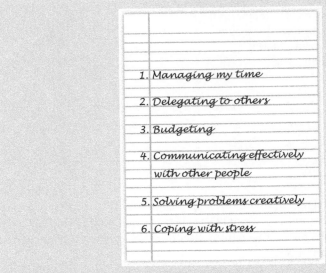

Figure 1.4   Annabelle's transferable skills

If reflection is thought of as a way to learn from experience, Annabelle has done that. The list of skills she identified clearly shows that she has thought purposefully about her experience of running her own business and has identified a number of skills that will be very useful to her. If, however, Annabelle was asked to submit her reflection as an assignment, what do you think the response to her list would be, or the response to her classmate who has drawn a picture? Such approaches are unlikely to be what the marking criteria for the assignment allocates marks to.

It is possible, however, for reflection to be a creative process. Writing in itself is a creative art and it is entirely possible for reflections to be presented in, or inspire, a wide range of creative forms such as a picture or a **storyboard**, a poem, a sculpture or even a play. Creativity is an excellent strategy to use when dealing with situations that evoke strong emotions, as it can help to overcome initial responses. This is considered in more detail in Chapter 5. It would be most unusual, however, for this type of creative reflection to be used within a nursing programme or even for revalidation. It is far more likely that the reflections that you and Annabelle need to produce will follow the accepted format of applying a tool, model or framework to highlight the reflective process.

REFLECTIVE TOOLS, MODELS AND FRAMEWORKS

ACTIVITY 1.4

Write down the names of any reflective tools, models or frameworks you have already heard of. Once you have done this, type 'reflective tools, models, frameworks' into an internet search engine.

How many different reflective tools, models or frameworks have you been able to identify?

Check the activity answers at the end of the chapter to see whether you found more than I did!

As you no doubt found in Activity 1.4, there are a large number of different reflective tools, models or frameworks. Whether these are called a tool, a model or a framework really does not make any difference; they are all designed to make the process of reflection easier. They do this by providing a specific structure to guide your reflection and help your 'thinking with a purpose'. Within this book, all these tools, models or frameworks will be referred to as 'models' in order to prevent confusion. Throughout this book, a number of frequently used models will be considered and examples will be given to provide illustrations as to how the model can be used and highlighting its benefits. Before thinking about individual models, however, it is necessary to think about something all models have in common – the six essential elements of reflection.

YOUR TOOLKIT FOR REFLECTION: THE SIX ESSENTIAL ELEMENTS

For a reflection to be effective, it requires the six essential elements of:

1. a critical incident;
2. a description;
3. an analysis;
4. an interpretation;
5. a perspective;
6. an action.

All models will help you to incorporate these six elements into your reflection. The best way to think about these six elements is as your toolkit for reflection. You are going to use them in a similar fashion to the way a skilled carpenter would use a tape measure, a hammer, a screwdriver, a saw and a plane to craft a window frame, except these tools will enable you to produce an effective reflection, applying whatever model you find most appropriate.

1. The critical incident

It is possible to reflect on any experience, but in order for a reflection to be useful, the experience chosen needs to be one you feel is important to you, plus you need to have a good reason for you to subject it to 'thinking with a purpose'. Such an experience is referred to as a 'critical incident'. In everyday discussion, the word 'critical' is often used to describe disapproving comments or judgements, and an incident is likely to be thought of as an occasion which probably was not positive. Even more worrying, if a patient is admitted to 'critical care', we think of this as meaning that things are not

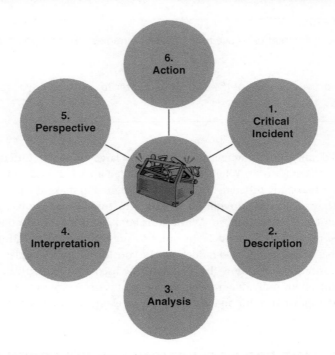

Figure 1.5 Your toolkit for reflection: the six essential elements

Source: Based on Jasper (2013).

going well for them. When talking about reflection, we need to forget these associa-tions, as they do not apply. In reflection, the term 'critical incident' is used to describe a specific experience that has meaning for the individual involved. This can, therefore, be any situation, and the individual could be directly involved in the experience because it is happening to them, or they might have observed it. As previously discussed, this could be either a positive or negative experience, meaning that it may have ended either in a way you felt happy about or made you worry. While you can reflect on either of these types of experience, as you can learn from both, it is important, as we have said, not only to use reflection for experiences that didn't go well. It is much better to take a more balanced approach and reflect on positive experiences, too. If you only ever reflect on things that don't go well, it is very easy to become disheartened about your ability. Always remember that reflection is also a way to think about the things you do well. This is important, as it will help you to understand why things went well, so you can work out how to repeat this experience and ensure consistently positive outcomes.

Deciding on what your critical incident will be is the first step in your reflection. Choosing a critical incident can, however, be quite tricky. You may find that an experi-ence that would be an excellent critical incident comes straight to mind. If it doesn't, it may be helpful to consider the reason why you are doing the reflection. This may be because you have been asked to do so, like Angus in Part A, or because you are going through the revalidation process, like Larry who we met at the start of the chapter. It could also be that you need to produce a reflection for an assignment, like Alex who we also met at the start of the chapter. Thinking about the reason for the reflection may provide further information as to what critical incident would be appropriate to choose.

For example, if your reflection is going to be submitted as an assignment, or is for revalidation, look at the guidelines, marking criteria and **learning outcomes** which have been provided.

Critical incidents are usually experiences that have occurred in the past, although it is possible to use reflection to prepare for things that you know are going to happen in the future, such as exams, interviews or upcoming placements.

When deciding on your critical incident, don't be overly ambitious; if you are, you will need to write lots of words to discuss all the topics you raise. When producing your first reflections, try to focus on just one or at most two main topics. If you look at Angus's reflection in Part A, you will see that while he was asked to reflect on his first day on placement, he actually focused on just one aspect of this and not on all the experiences he had.

2. The description

In order to start thinking with a purpose, or reflecting, you need to clearly describe the experience you are going to focus on. It is important to describe what happened very carefully, making sure that you include all the relevant points. There are four words that are very helpful when you are writing your description:

- Who?
- What?
- Where?
- When?

These will help you to ensure that you include the important aspects in your description, so you provide a clear overview.

3. The analysis

In its simplest form, analysis is breaking something down to its essential parts and making a judgement based on the information this provides. To do this successfully, throughout your reflection you need to take a step back from the situation, so you can consider the relevant topics **objectively**. Being objective is a very important aspect of reflection, as you need to consider your actions and possibly those of any other individuals involved in the experience without any emotions that might cloud your ability to come to a sound judgement. In the analysis section there are another two words which are very useful:

- Why?
- How?

Using 'Why?' and 'How?' will help you to make a judgement based on the information you have obtained and suggest some possible conclusions. Using these two words will help you to ask good questions such as:

- Why do I feel how I do about this experience?
- How did the experience make the others involved feel?

- Why did I do what I did?
- How did the others involved act?
- How do I know I took the correct course of action?
- Why did things happen as they did in this experience?

These sorts of questions will help you to gain insight into the experience and start to understand why you, and any others involved, acted in the way they did.

The analysis section represents a very important step towards becoming a reflective practitioner, as it will help you to become aware of the reasons for your actions. It is possible that this may make you feel uneasy as you review experiences that may have been difficult and realise the consequences of your actions. Accepting responsibility for your actions and being honest are important features of the professional practice of a nurse. Being honest in your reflections will enable you to combine the insight that reflection brings with accurate nursing knowledge and skills, thus ensuring that you are a safe and effective practitioner.

The possible conclusions you come to as a result of your analysis may make you think that you have done the wrong thing or that you are presenting yourself in a negative fashion. This is not something to worry about; again, you are acting in a professional manner by doing this. It is, in fact, this process that will enable you to learn from your experience and not repeat mistakes in the future.

4. The interpretation

Once you have analysed your experience and come to some possible conclusions, interpreting this will enable you to gain a deeper understanding of the experience. By interpreting aspects of your experience, you will explore the different components of it even further. The interpretation of an experience is where you consider what happened with reference to other, additional information. What this means is that you think very carefully about the reasons you and others acted in the ways you did and, using other information, make suggestions as to potential explanations for this. Remember the importance of being objective, taking a step back and ensuring that your emotions do not cloud your judgement. Reflection is not a process of criticising yourself and others, but one of learning from your experience.

Once again, this process may make you feel uncomfortable, as it may involve you in considering topics you could have previously ignored. This is all part of your journey to becoming a reflective practitioner. What is important is that you think about your experience in terms of what you can do better in the future.

5. Another perspective

When you think about your experience from another perspective, what you are doing is looking at your experience, but not with your eyes. You are trying to see it from an alternative viewpoint. This can be very difficult, and a good way to start doing this is by talking to others about your experience. Your fellow students, **practice supervisor**, **practice assessor** or lecturer are good people to do this with, as they are likely to have some understanding of the experience and will be very happy to share their thoughts with you. By doing this, you will gain their perspective on the experience, so you will be able to see it through their eyes. Seeing an experience through the eyes of another person enables you to become aware of your specific view of the world, which can help to highlight the things you take for granted and do not question. This is, therefore, an excellent way to gain an objective view of an experience, because if you talk to others about it, the experience is no longer being considered just from your personal perspective.

If you are unable to talk to others about an experience, you can still put yourself in their shoes and think about what their thoughts and feelings could be. Try to imagine what they would say to you about the conclusions you have come to. It is often the case that we judge ourselves very harshly; thinking an experience through from another perspective may enable you to see your actions more positively.

6. Action

Action is the final tool in your kit and possibly the most important. As we have already said, reflection is a process of learning and the result of this learning is to be able to base future actions on the knowledge gained. It is possible that this knowledge may relate to specific nursing theory or skill, or could relate to more personal topics, such as your attitude.

The action you highlight depends on all of the thinking you have done about your experience using your other five tools. What is really important to remember is that reflection is actually all about *you*. While other individuals may have been involved in your experience, it is only possible for you to be responsible for changing your future actions. While we might see the need for change in others, this will only happen when they see this need for themselves.

ACTIVITY 1.5

In a small qualitative research study, Stirling (2015) considered the views of students and lecturers relating to the use of reflection in nurse education. The paper clearly highlights both the benefits of reflection and the barriers to its use, and makes clear suggestions for improvement.

Read the article and consider how you can relate the findings to your reflections.

Stirling, L. (2015) Students' and tutors' perceptions of the use of reflection in post-registration nurse education. *Community Practitioner*, April, 38–41.

There is no definitive answer to this activity as the question is based on your own reflection.

MAKING A GOOD START WHEN REFLECTING

You are now nearly at the point of being able to undertake a reflection of your own. There is just one further important issue we need to consider.

Throughout the chapter so far there has been discussion of reflective models and that there are many different models designed to help you. In order to produce an effective reflection, and especially if it is going to be formally submitted – for example, as an assignment – you need to apply a reflective model. When starting to use reflection, Borton's model (1970) is a good one to use and it will help you to make a good start. It is very straightforward to apply; as you can see from Figure 1.6, the model is actually made up of just three questions.

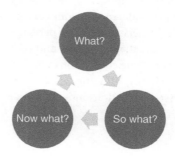

Figure 1.6   Borton's model (1970)

The simplicity of Borton's model makes it particularly useful for novice reflective practitioners, although it can also be used at different levels as you become more experienced, as we will discuss in Chapter 2. The structure of Borton's model is very helpful in learning from experience and translating your experience into action. As seen in Figure 1.6, the model contains all of the six essential elements of reflection:

- What? contains elements 1 and 2 – the critical incident and description.
- So what? contains elements 3, 4 and 5 – the analysis, interpretation and viewing from another perspective.
- What now? contains element 6 – the action.

Possibly, what makes this model the best to use for your first reflections is its structure. Having just three questions means that it is easy to remember.

If you look at Part A, you will see that Angus used Borton's model (1970) to structure his reflection on his first day in placement.

ACTIVITY 1.6

Read Angus's reflection in Part A and think about how you could use Borton's model (1970) to structure a reflection of your own.

There is no definitive answer to this activity. However, you will find hints and tips as to how you can do this in Chapter 2.

CONCLUSION

Reflection has a fundamental role in nursing, as it enables learning from experience, which ensures that patients receive the best care possible. By being a reflective practitioner, a nurse also learns about themselves and can apply this knowledge to their future actions.

There are many reflective tools, models or frameworks, all of which are designed to make the process of reflection easier. Borton's model (1970) is an excellent model for the novice reflector, as not only is it simple, straightforward to use and easy to remember, it is also effective in supporting learning from experience and translating this into action.

GOING FURTHER

Esterhuizen, P. (2019) *Reflective Practice in Nursing* (4th edn). London: SAGE. This book provides a clear and straightforward introduction to reflection with a range of activities to increase your confidence.

Somerville, D. and Keeling, J. (2004) A practical approach to promote reflective practice within nursing. *Nursing Times*, 100(12): 42–5. While this article is more than ten years old, it presents an excellent overview of the topic, which remains relevant. Some myths surrounding reflective practice are dispelled and good examples of the benefits of reflection are highlighted.

Understanding reflective practice. Go to: https://journals.rcni.com/doi/abs/10.7748/ns.30.36.34.s44. This web-link provides practical guidance to help practitioners use reflective models to write reflective accounts.

ANSWERS TO ACTIVITIES

Activity 1.1

There are many answers to this question, some of which will be personal to you, so you may have some that are not on the list of possible answers. When you are next with other nurses or nursing students, ask them what they think and compare notes.

Possible answers: to make sure they provide the best patient care; to understand themselves; to develop nursing knowledge; to learn from experience; to pass assignments; to revalidate; to decide what they need to know more about; to decide how they will act in similar situations; to work out what went well and what they want to improve on; to decide on goals you want to achieve.

Activity 1.4

My search resulted in a total of 35 different reflective tools, models and frameworks, but you may have found more. If you compare the ones you have found, you will see that many are very similar and they all contain the six essential elements of reflection.

GLOSSARY

cognitive   Connected with thinking or conscious mental processes.

interchangeably   Can be used in place of each other.

learning outcomes   Statements identifying the knowledge, skill or attitude a learner possesses after completing a learning activity.

mindful Constant vigilance against unskilful actions and negative attitudes that could cloud your judgement.

Nursing and Midwifery Council (NMC) The regulator for Nursing and Midwifery in the United Kingdom.

objectively Not influenced by personal feelings, views or prejudice – based on facts.

practice assessor A nurse who assesses a student's overall performance for their practice learning.

practice supervisor A registered health or social care professional who supervises nursing students on placements.

reflection Thinking with a purpose.

reflective Being thoughtful.

reflective discussion The process of talking with another person about a reflection and the spoken reflection itself.

reflective practice Thinking about an experience and learning from it.

reflective practitioner A nurse (or other healthcare professional) who uses what they have learnt from experience to develop their knowledge and deliver the best care possible.

reflective processes Specifically structured methods that enable new actions to be based on learning gained from experience.

reflexive Being thoughtful.

reflexive writing The process of writing a reflection and the written reflection itself.

retrospective contemplation Thinking about something that happened in the past.

revalidation The process that allows a registered nurse to maintain their registration with the NMC, which demonstrates their continued ability to practise safely and effectively.

storyboard A sequence of drawings, usually with some dialogue, which tell a story.

REFERENCES

Borton, T. (1970) *Reach, Touch and Teach*. London: Hutchinson.

Department of Health (DH) (2012) *Compassion in Practice*. London: Department of Health.

Glaze, J. (2002) Stages in coming to terms with reflection: student advanced nurse practitioners' perceptions of their reflective journals. *Journal of Advanced Nursing*, 37(3): 265–72.

Jasper, M. (2013) *Beginning Reflective Practice* (2nd edn). Andover: Cengage Learning EMEA.

Johns, C. (2017) *Becoming a Reflective Practitioner*. Chichester: Wiley-Blackwell.

Nursing and Midwifery Council (NMC) (2018) *The Code*. London: NMC.

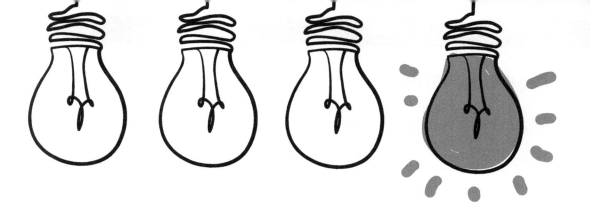

A FIRST REFLECTION

CATHERINE DELVES-YATES

2

I am really not sure how to start out writing a reflection – I know I need to use a model, but which one, and how do I put my experience on paper?

Theo Ha, nursing student, adult field

I have lots of experiences I would like to reflect on for revalidation and I have been reading about reflective models. I think everything is going well until I try to start writing, then I am stuck . . .

Jenny Esoh, registered nurse, mental health field

INTRODUCTION

While the primary activity we undertake when reflecting is 'thinking with a purpose', as Theo and Jenny tell us at the start of this chapter, we often need to make a written record of our reflections. Working out how it is best to turn our thinking about an experience, which may be jumbled and multifaceted, into logical, clear and understandable writing, can be daunting.

Taking a step-by-step approach, this chapter will develop what we considered in Chapter 1, and outline strategies you can use to develop your thinking with a purpose about an experience into a written reflection. First, we will consider exactly what elements your written reflection needs to contain in order to be effective. Following this, you will be introduced to a simple strategy you can use to 'get writing'. Lastly, the chapter will end with a plan for writing a reflection that you can adapt and follow. This plan will assist you to ensure that your reflection demonstrates careful consideration (or thinking with a purpose) relating to the topic or topics you have focused on.

Throughout this chapter, relevant links will be made to Angus's reflection in Part A. Angus's reflection will be reviewed and refined in this and the following chapters of this part of the book. The aim of this is to provide you with an example for how your reflection can be developed from your initial thoughts.

CHAPTER AIMS

This chapter will enable you to:

- capture all of the six essential elements in your reflection;
- understand and utilise Goodman's levels of reflection;
- practise 'free writing' to get your reflection started;
- apply Borton's (1970) model of reflection;
- develop a personalised plan for writing an effective reflection.

CAPTURING THE SIX 'ESSENTIAL ELEMENTS' OF A REFLECTION

As we discussed in Chapter 1, even though there are many different models of reflection, they all have one thing in common. All models contain the six essential elements, or what you can think of as your reflection toolkit, as shown in Figure 2.1.

Thinking of the

- critical incident
- description
- analysis
- interpretation
- perspective
- action

as your reflection toolkit and identifying where each element is positioned within the reflective model you are planning to use is an excellent starting point for a written reflection.

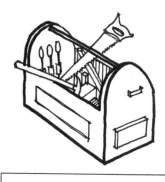 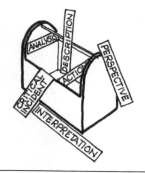

A toolkit contains all of the essential tools we need to do a specific job	When you reflect you can use a toolkit, but rather than saws, hammers and planes, you have the six essential elements

Figure 2.1   Your toolkit for reflection: the six essential elements

Source: Based on Jasper (2013).

In this way, you can identify a number of questions or points to consider as you work through your chosen model. While this may seem daunting at the moment, it is actually far easier than you might think.

ACTIVITY 2.1

Refer to Part A and read the reflection that Angus wrote using Borton's (1970) model following his first day in placement.

- How many of the essential elements you can find in what Angus wrote?

Check the activity answers at the end of the chapter to see if we agree.

HOW THE SIX 'ESSENTIAL ELEMENTS' HELP

The six 'essential elements' can be used as helpful prompts to make sure that your reflection not only describes your experience, but assists you to demonstrate in your writing that you have thought about it in a **systematic** fashion, demonstrating both breadth and depth of thinking. As we have discussed, reflection can be thought of as being rather like an onion, in that it has many layers. The key to becoming a truly reflective nurse who delivers mindful practice is to peel away the layers of the onion. This will enable you to go from the simple approach of a novice who is sitting on the skin of the onion and 'doing reflection' to the more complex approach of 'being reflective' at the very centre of the onion.

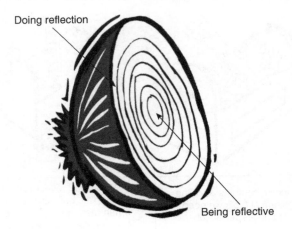

Doing reflection

Being reflective

Figure 2.2   Reflection as an onion

Source: Adapted from Johns (2013) © *Becoming a Reflective Practitioner* (4th edn). By kind permission of John Wiley & Sons.

Thinking widely and deeply is an integral aspect of the journey from a novice reflector to a mindful practitioner. Part of becoming more experienced at reflecting and writing your thoughts down is to think critically and write in an academic fashion. Writing and strategies to further develop your critical thinking ability in your reflections are covered in greater detail in Chapter 3. Before we consider critical thinking, a good way to start to develop your ability to reflect is to understand the difference between how we talk generally and how we write and express thoughts in an academic or formal piece of writing.

ACTIVITY 2.2

Refer to the Angus Plumb case study in Part A and read the section *Hi! Angus here!* which is Angus talking. Then read *Angus's reflection* on writing his thoughts down in a more formal way.

• Can you notice any differences?

Check the activity answers at the end of the chapter to see if we agree.

Generally, when we speak we use informal language, but when we write our language is far more formal. A good way to consider this is to think about what you said when you last spoke to a friend, or even sent them a text. It is unlikely that you used the same style of language as you are reading in this book. We customise our use of language to fit each specific situation, no matter whether it is spoken or written. Think back to the last conversation you had with a friend or relative; it was likely to have been very different from how you hear the newsreader speaking when you listen to the news. As you work to develop your ability to reflect and, just as importantly, to make a written record of your reflection, you will become more proficient at using the appropriate style of writing.

HOW MUCH EXPERIENCE . . . ?

You may be reading this book as a nursing student with very little nursing experience who thinks of themselves as a nursing novice, or you may be reading this book as a registered nurse with a great deal of nursing experience who is viewed as an expert. Reflection has a role to play in both cases, as it is essential in highlighting knowledge gained from experience. By applying knowledge gained from experience to the care you provide, you will be able to assess new situations and deliver effective interventions. Thus, while reflection is key in the journey from novice to expert nurse, it is also fundamental in ensuring that an expert nurse remains confident and competent in their own expertise.

USING MODELS

As we have previously discussed, there is a wide range of models that can be used to assist you to reflect. Many of these comprise a series of headings for sections that you can use to develop your reflection, as we have already seen in the reflection that Angus wrote using Borton's model (1970). A model which takes a slightly different approach was developed by Goodman (1984) who developed a model outlining that there are three levels of reflection that can be achieved. Figure 2.3 identifies what Goodman (1984) suggested each level is composed of.

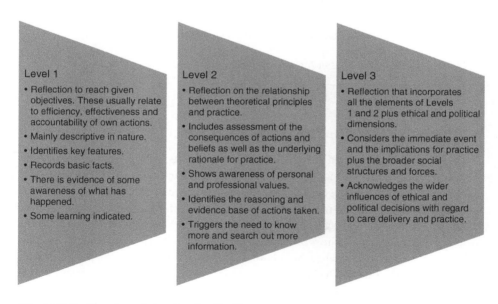

Figure 2.3 Goodman's levels of reflection

Source: Adapted by kind permission of Springer Nature. Goodman (1984) © Reflection and teacher education: A case study and theoretical analysis, *Interchange*.

If we review Figure 2.3, it is possible to summarise that Goodman's (1984) Level 1 is mainly descriptive, with the reflection reading rather like a story. This may well be the case with the first few reflections you write. Level 1 reflections present a good descriptive account of the experience and consider feelings, but do not go any deeper than this. As you get more used to writing in a reflexive way, become familiar with the model of reflection you are using and get better at questioning your thoughts and actions (critical thinking), your reflections will start to consider the relationship between theoretical principles (your knowledge base) and practice. At this point your work will become more **analytical**, identifying learning and coming to conclusions about actions which can be transferred to other situations. This is reflection at Goodman's (1984) Level 2. As you develop your reflexive thinking even further, the breadth and depth of your consideration will increase, to include, for example, important issues such as ethical and political aspects. At this stage you will have achieved Goodman's Level 3 and be well on your way to becoming a truly reflexive practitioner.

In this way, therefore, Goodman's (1984) levels are helpful when deciding what you need to consider in a reflection, as they can be used as a list of the elements you need to include. This is even more important if the reflection is for an assignment during an academic course, as the expectation will be that your reflections develop during the course and you will achieve Goodman's (1984) Level 3.

ACTIVITY 2.3

Read Angus's reflection in Part A.

* Which of Goodman's levels do you think he achieves?

Check the activity answers at the end of the chapter to see if we agree.

GETTING STARTED: THE FIRST STEPS

The best way to become good at reflection, like many things, is to practise. Think back to when you first tried to ride a bicycle, skateboard or put on roller-skates. It took practice to stop you feeling 'wobbly' or falling over, and even more practice to be able to go in the direction you wanted in a graceful manner, thereby becoming an expert. Reflection is just the same.

The first step when writing a reflection is to decide what experience is going to be the focus of your reflection and, in writing, describe it. As we outlined in Chapter 1, it is possible to reflect on any experience, but in order for a reflection to be useful, the experience chosen needs to be one you feel is important to you. Such an experience is referred to as a 'critical incident'. For Angus, the critical incident was his first day on placement, but if you refer to his reflection, he did not try to cover everything that happened on that day, but instead selected a specific issue. This is a very sensible approach, as unless you want your reflection to be many pages long (and often this will not be possible, as when you are reflecting for the purpose of an assessment, you will be given a maximum word allowance), it is best to limit yourself to focus on only one issue.

The second step is to choose which reflective model you are going to use. For the rest of this chapter we will refer to Borton's (1970) model, which is an excellent model to use when you are starting reflection, and is the one that Angus used.

As Jenny mentioned at the start of the chapter, however, actually starting to put words down on paper relating to an experience can often be a stumbling block.

Figure 2.4 provides a very good tip that will help Jenny, and you, to start writing.

Write a description of your critical incident for 5–15 minutes without stopping to read what you have written.

- Imagine you are talking to yourself on paper.
- Write quickly and don't worry about your spelling or grammar.

If you wander off the topic, just bring yourself back to the focus of your reflection.

- When the time is up, read through what you have written to identify the useful words, phrases, thoughts and ideas.
- Develop this into your description.

Figure 2.4   **Tips to help you start writing**

Source: Based on free writing (Elbow, 1973).

It is always very much easier to write if you already have a few words on your paper. Even if, at this stage, you are not certain that they are the correct words or even in the correct order, the more words you can have on your paper, the less off-putting writing will become.

ACTIVITY 2.4

Follow the tips identified in Figure 2.4 and 'free write' the description of your critical incident.

Remember that you should write without reading what you have already written for 5-15 minutes and only then start to refine what you have written.

There is no definitive answer to this activity as the question is based on your own writing.

NEXT STEPS IN YOUR REFLECTION

As we have already highlighted, in order to construct a reflection, we are going to apply Borton's (1970) model. The simplicity of his model makes it particularly useful for novice reflective practitioners, although it can also be used at all of Goodman's (1984) levels as you become more experienced. The structure of Borton's (1970) model is very helpful in learning from experience and translating the knowledge gained from your experience into action. It contains all of the six essential elements of reflection and possibly, most importantly, its structure, just three questions, means that it is easy to remember.

As we have discussed, in order to make a reflection effective, it needs to contain each of the six essential elements. Figure 2.5 shows where each of these fit in Borton's (1970) model.

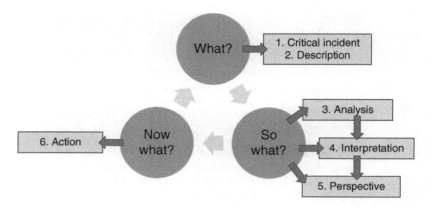

Figure 2.5   The six essential elements: what goes where in Borton's (1970) model?

A PLAN

Table 2.1 shows you how Borton's (1970) model can be used to contain all the elements we have discussed in this chapter so far. This provides you with a plan you can follow to write your reflection. You can customise this plan, as you may decide that not all aspects are relevant to the reflection you are writing, or you may decide to add some additional ones. The choice is yours because, as we have said previously, a reflection is really about you, and so, even if we are all using the same plan, what you develop will be just as unique as you are.

Table 2.1   How you can use Borton's (1970) model

Borton's (1970) Model	Remember
What? Essential elements included in this stage: • critical incident; • description.	Focus on just one aspect of your experience so you can consider this issue in detail, rather than trying to consider lots of issues and not achieving any depth in your reflection.
This is the description of your critical incident. Here you write an overview of your experience describing: • What was the **context** for the experience? • Why is this experience important to you? • What happened? • How you were involved? • What exactly did you do? • What were your thoughts and feelings? • How did you respond to what happened?	Make sure that your description is clear, so that the reader fully understands your experience. You are unlikely to be able to write a clear description on the first attempt at writing your experience down, so keep reading what you have written and refine it, until it says exactly what you want it to. At this point it can be useful to ask a friend to read what you have written and give you some feedback.

Borton's (1970) Model	Remember

So what?

Essential elements included in this stage:

- analysis;
- interpretation;
- perspective.

This is where you break the experience down so you can question:

- What was important in this experience?
- What were your thoughts and feelings during the experience?
- What theory relates to your experience?
- What went well?
- What could have gone better?
- What were the consequences of your actions and beliefs?
- Does the experience make you rethink your actions and beliefs?
- What did the experience teach you?
- How do your personal and professional values relate to the experience?
- What would you do differently if you were faced with a similar situation - what would be the different actions or approaches you could take?
- What is the significance of what happened?
- What else do you need to consider to understand more fully what happened?
- What sense can you make of this experience?
- How did this experience influence or change you?

In this stage, the aim is to clearly demonstrate that you have carefully considered your experience and thought about the relationship between theoretical principles and practice.

Your consideration needs to include discussion relating to the consequences of your actions and beliefs and, if relevant, those of any others involved.

You need to provide evidence that you are aware of both your personal and professional values.

To produce an effective reflection which achieves Goodman's Level 2 or 3, this section needs to use references to support the statements you are making. This will enable you to identify the reasoning behind and the evidence base of the actions you took.

To achieve Goodman's Level 3, you also need to consider the broader social structures and forces plus the wider influences of ethical and political decisions with regard to care delivery and practice.

What now?

Essential element included in this stage: action

This where you put things back together, the **synthesis**, and relate this experience to your future considering:

- What do you need to do now?
- What do I need to learn following my experience?
- How are you going to do this?

It is important in this section to demonstrate that you understand the need to know more and the actions you are going to take to achieve this.

You are now very nearly at the stage where you are ready to write your reflection using Borton's (1970) model. There is just one more useful activity you need to undertake which will make you confident that you are aware of everything you need to include to produce an effective reflection.

ACTIVITY 2.5

Read Angus's reflection in Part A.

- What parts of the plan in Table 2.1 could Angus have added to his reflection to make it more effective?

Write down what you think he could have added and then check the answer at the end of the chapter to see if we agree.

I think what makes a really good nurse is that they realise they need to keep learning. They may repeat the same activities with lots of different patients, but because the patients are individuals, they will need to do it a little differently each time. Learning from experience, and also continuing to learn from all new experiences is how a nurse can be sure the care they deliver remains good.

Lizzie Evans, patient

As Lizzie tells us, reflecting on critical incidents and new experiences is an excellent way to constantly develop your knowledge and ensure that you keep your skills up to date. While the fundamental theory you will learn or, maybe, have learnt many years ago, is likely to remain applicable to the care you deliver, due to advances in technology how you actually carry out a skill may change. This makes it even more important that in your reflections you identify the reasoning behind the actions you take and the evidence base supporting them. Doing this will help you to understand how you know what you are doing is correct. This can be one of the most challenging aspects of writing an effective reflection, and is covered in more detail in Chapter 3.

ACTIVITY 2.6

Using Table 2.1 as a plan, develop the ideas you 'free wrote' in Activity 2.4 into a reflection. In order to ensure that this activity doesn't take you too much time to complete, aim to write no more than 1,000 words in total.

Review and rewrite what you have written until you are happy that it clearly outlines your experience and demonstrates that you have thought carefully about the topic or topics it highlighted. Writing is hard work, and it takes a great deal of time to craft an end result you can be proud of. Once you have achieved this, share it with a friend and ask them to provide you with feedback on what you have written.

There is no definitive answer for this activity as it is based on your own experience.

CONCLUSION

Reflection is key in the journey from novice to expert nurse and fundamental in ensuring that an expert nurse remains confident in their own expertise. Writing a reflection, however, especially if this is for an assessment or revalidation, can seem daunting. Do not let this put you off, as there are many strategies that can help with this process.

While there are many different models of reflection, they all contain the six essential elements of a critical incident, description, analysis, interpretation, perspective and action. In order for your reflection to be effective, you need to consider all of these elements in relation to your experience. This will demonstrate to those who read your work that you have thought in a systematic fashion with breadth and depth of thinking. This is important not only to ensure that you learn as much as possible from your experience, but it will assist you to produce a reflection that is of a good standard when you are submitting your work for a formal purpose. Achieving this good standard can take a great deal of practice. Reflection is a skill, so remember that the more you reflect, the better you will become at it.

There are many tips that can help you while you practise reflection. Goodman's (1984) levels of reflection will assist you to produce a reflection that achieves the required academic standard. Starting your writing with the 'free writing' technique will enable you to get those first and often difficult words on paper. In addition to this, using a model that is appropriate for how much reflection you have undertaken will also ensure success.

Reflecting on critical incidents is an excellent way to develop your nursing knowledge and skill, and all the time you practise you will be developing into a truly reflective practitioner.

GOING FURTHER

Coward, M. (2018) Reflection and professional learning. *Nursing Management*. doi: 10.7748/nm.2018.e1752. This is an excellent article that uses a number of activities in order to assist you to consider the purpose of reflecting beyond professional requirements, the influence of our experiences on who we are and what we learn, the value of protected time to think and the benefits of reflecting for personal development.

McKinnon, J. (2016) *Reflection for Nursing Life*. London: Routledge. A very readable textbook that uses stories to help you to consider your own practice by identifying your strengths and weaknesses, and then provides tips to overcome them.

The lasting value of reflection. Go to: www.youtube.com/watch?v=G1bgdwC_m-Y. This weblink will take you to an interesting and informative TED talk considering the lasting value of reflection.

──────── ANSWERS TO ACTIVITIES ────────

Activity 2.1

Table 2.2   Essential elements in Angus's reflection

Angus's reflection	The six elements
What?	
Yesterday was the first day of my first ever clinical placement.	This is the critical incident.
I really enjoyed it, but I feel that there is so very much to learn and I am worried that I am never going to get the hang of it. I feel that everyone else knows so much more than me and I am finding it hard to be confident about my ability at the moment.	This is the description.
So what?	
If I don't know enough, I might do the wrong thing. This could result in a patient not getting the right treatment. This does worry me, as we have had lots of sessions about the importance of *The Code* (NMC, 2018).	This is the analysis.
Thinking a bit more about this in particular, remembering how I felt on my first day when I was a volunteer teacher in the school in Africa, I felt the same.	This is the interpretation.
Until now, I had forgotten that it took me a couple of weeks to feel that I had a little bit of an idea as to what I needed to do.	This is the perspective.
Now what?	
I need to make sure that I only do the things I know are correct and if I am not sure, I have got to ask and not feel that I am being a pain if I need to do this. My mentor is there to guide me. She is great at this, so I need to work closely with her. If I do this, I won't feel so out of my depth.	All of this section is the action.
I need to give myself a bit of time and not expect that I can go into a new situation, be an expert and feel comfortable straight away.	

Activity 2.2

The difference is the level of formality. Angus's choice of words, style and the way the words he uses are put together differ between the two sections. When Angus is speaking, he is being much less formal and more personal in the terms he uses than what he writes in his reflection. You can also see that he is being less formal in how he applies the rules of grammar. For example, in his speaking he says 'I'm', but when he writes he doesn't use such abbreviations, but writes all the words out in full.

Activity 2.3

Angus's reflection

In the extract below, the text that appears in italics is taken directly from the description of Goodman's (1984) levels in Figure 2.3, so you can see exactly which aspects Angus achieves.

Within this reflection Angus is concentrating on *the efficiency, effectiveness and account-ability of his own actions*. What he has written is *mainly descriptive in nature*. He clearly *identifies key features* and *records basic facts*. There *is some awareness of what has hap-pened, and some learning is indicated*. So, he has clearly achieved Goodman's (1984) Level 1.

If we look at the elements required for Level 2, Angus hasn't made any comment on *the relationship between theoretical principles and practice*. He does make some *assessment of the* potential *consequences of* his *actions*, but does not develop this to consider *beliefs* or *the underlying rationale for* his *practice*. Angus doesn't clearly *demonstrate aware-ness of personal and professional values* or *identify the reasoning and evidence base of actions taken*, but his consideration does trigger *the need to know more and search out more information*.

As Angus hasn't achieved all of the aspects of Level 2, he cannot achieve Level 3, as the starting point for Level 3 is that the reflection *incorporates all the elements of levels 1 and 2*.

So the answer is that Angus's reflection achieves Goodman's (1984) Level 1, which for a first reflection is exactly what is expected.

Activity 2.5

Table 2.3   How Angus's reflection can be improved

Angus's reflection	How Angus's reflection can be improved
What?	This is the description of Angus's critical incident, so here he needs to describe what the context for his experience was, why it was important, what happened, how he was involved, what he did, what his thoughts and feelings were and how he responded to what happened.
Yesterday was the first day of my first ever clinical placement. I really enjoyed it, but I feel that there is so very much to learn and I am worried that I am never going to get the hang of it. I feel that everyone else knows so much more than me and I am finding it hard to be confident about my ability at the moment.	Angus was very sensible to focus on only one aspect of his first day on placement, so his critical incident relates to his lack of knowledge, which is making him feel unconfident. He has done a good job to describe it here. He has concentrated on his concerns, rather than giving a very detailed description of everything that happened. He has used his words well, so we understand exactly what the topic is that he is reflecting on.
So what?	In this section, Angus needs to include the essential elements of analysis, interpretation and perspective. Here he needs to question what was important, what his thoughts and feelings were, what theory relates to his experience, what went well and what could have gone better, what were the consequences of his actions or beliefs, whether the experience made him rethink his actions and beliefs, what he learnt, how his personal and professional values relate to the experience, what he would do differently next time, what is the significance of what happened, what else he needs to consider to understand more fully what happened, what sense he can make of the experience and how the experience influenced or changed him.
If I don't know enough I might do the wrong thing. This could result in a patient not getting the right treatment. This does worry me, as we have had lots of sessions about the importance of *The Code* (NMC, 2018).	

(Continued)

Table 2.3   (Continued)

Angus's reflection	How Angus's reflection can be improved
Thinking a bit more about this in particular, remembering how I felt on my first day when I was a volunteer teacher in the school in Africa, I felt the same. Until now, I had forgotten that it took me a couple of weeks to feel that I had a little bit of an idea as to what I needed to do.	Again, here he did a good job at producing his first reflection. He questioned what was important – that he might do the wrong thing, considered his feelings, related theory to his experience – *The Code* (NMC, 2018) – and thought about how he could make sense of the experience by considering how he felt on his first day as a volunteer teacher. These are all a good start and he achieved Goodman's Level 1. However, he could have provided more evidence of his thinking about the relationship between theoretical principles and practice by relating his discussion to more relevant evidence, using references to support what he was saying, and to provide further evidence that he was aware of his personal and professional values. If he had done this, he would have achieved Goodman's Level 2, as he would have identified the reasoning behind and the evidence base supporting what he was considering. To achieve Goodman's Level 3, Angus needed to consider the wider influences of ethical and political decisions with regard to his experience. So, for example, he could have considered whether having more nursing staff for him to work with (as a political perspective) and whether it is acceptable for patients to be cared for by nursing students with very little experience (as an ethical perspective). Again, all of this discussion needed to be supported by relevant evidence.
Now what?	In this section, Angus needs to consider the final essential element of action, showing that he has considered what he said in the previous sections in relation to possible experiences in the future.
I need to make sure that I only do the things I know are correct and, if I am not sure, I have got to ask and not feel that I am being a pain if I need to do this. My mentor is there to guide me. She is great at this, so I need to work closely with her. If I do this, I won't feel so out of my depth.	Angus did a good job here, too. He clearly identified what he needed to do now, what he had learnt from his experience and how he was going to use this experience in the future.
I need to give myself a bit of time and not expect that I can go into a new situation, be an expert and feel comfortable straight away.	

GLOSSARY

analytical   Investigating and being critical.

context   The setting and the background.

synthesis   Combining elements.

systematic   Applying a comprehensive, methodical and logical approach.

REFERENCES

Borton, T. (1970) *Reach, Touch and Teach*. London: Hutchinson.

Elbow, P. (1973) *Writing Without Teachers*. New York: Oxford University Press.

Goodman, J. (1984) Reflection and teacher education: a case study and theoretical analysis. *Interchanges*, 15: 9–26.

Jasper, M. (2013) *Beginning Reflective Practice* (2nd edn). Andover: Cengage Learning EMEA.

Johns, C. (2013) *Becoming a Reflective Practitioner*. Chichester: Wiley-Blackwell.

Nursing and Midwifery Council (NMC) (2018) *The Code*. London: NMC.

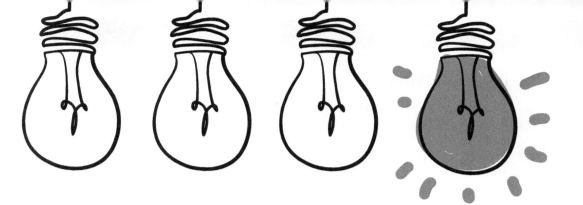

THINKING CRITICALLY

CATHERINE DELVES-YATES

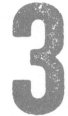

> In my feedback for my last reflection I was told I needed to show in my writing that I was thinking critically . . . I don't understand exactly what that means. As I see it, 'thinking' means considering a topic carefully and 'being critical' means asking questions. I am doing that.
>
> **Faith Boyo, nursing student, adult field**

> I find critical thinking really hard. I need to know how to do this more effectively.
>
> **Oscar Riley, registered nurse, mental health field**

INTRODUCTION

It is possible that many of us may share Faith's confusion as to exactly what is meant by the term 'thinking critically'. Faith has made a good try at working out what she should be doing, but she has actually missed a very important difference between everyday thinking, which is what she is describing, and critical thinking, which is what she needs to do.

Naturally, when we think, the judgements we make are often uncritical, because they are based on personal bias, self-interest or irrational emotions. So, when we undertake everyday thinking we are not **objective**. It is objectivity that is the key to becoming a critical thinker. The need to be objective is the reason critical thinking is a skill, which, like riding a bicycle, you have to work on to acquire and improve. In addition to this, writing is hard work. So, to produce a good written reflection containing both clear writing and critical thinking, it is necessary to think about the topic in great detail, ask questions, come to logical objective conclusions, and then review and refine your work. Normally, it is necessary to do the review and refining stage more than once. Producing a good piece of written work is much more like running a marathon than it is a sprint. The key to success is not to give up – just like a marathon runner, both you, and Faith, have to keep working at it.

In this chapter, we will review and refine Angus's reflection in Part A in order to show how it could be further developed to demonstrate critical thinking. Following this process will assist you to understand how you can make your reflections demonstrate critical thinking. As Oscar says at the start of the chapter, this is a difficult task, but there are ways to do it effectively. Producing an effective reflection is achieved by working through a series of stages. These stages start with initial thoughts and free writing, progress through organising the reflection to follow a reflective model and finally crafting it into an effective, critical piece of writing. We have already achieved some of the steps involved in these stages in Chapters 1 and 2. By the end of this chapter, we won't quite have completed our marathon, but we will be approaching the home straight!

CHAPTER AIMS

This chapter will enable you to:

- understand what critical thinking is;
- appreciate why you need to think critically when reflecting;
- realise the importance of considering relevant evidence;
- demonstrate critical thinking in your writing.

WHAT IS CRITICAL THINKING?

As Faith demonstrated at the start of this chapter, understanding exactly what is meant by the term 'critical thinking' can be difficult and it is easy to become confused as to how it differs from everyday thinking. An experience you may have had, which simply demonstrates the difference between everyday thinking and critical thinking, is when you come home, tired and hungry, following a long a busy shift caring for patients.

You are desperate for something to eat, but as you have to get up early for another shift tomorrow, you don't want to spend any time cooking. In your food cupboard you have a family-sized bar of chocolate, a loaf of bread and a tin of baked beans. Thinking about what you can have to eat, the options are the big bar of chocolate or baked beans on toast. As is shown in Figure 3.1, it is possible to make your choice using either everyday thinking or critical thinking.

Everyday thinking...
"Yeah! Great big bar of chocolate for supper. Yummy. I love chocolate and there is loads of it in that bar. Goody!!"

Choice – bar of chocolate

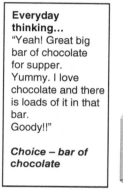
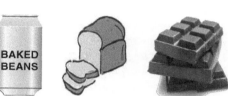

Critical thinking...
"A big bar of chocolate, or baked beans on toast for supper? As much as I love chocolate, I know that baked beans on toast is far more nutritious."

Choice – beans on toast

Figure 3.1   Everyday thinking vs. critical thinking

In Figure 3.1, the choice of the bar of chocolate, resulting from the everyday thinking, is not an objective one; it is an emotional choice, based on the love of chocolate. While the choice of beans on toast is as a result of a very simplified version of critical thinking, it does actually involve applying evidence-based knowledge to a specific situation in order to come to a sound conclusion. You will see later in the chapter that this is an important aspect of critical thinking.

As we discussed when we talked about a critical incident in Chapter 1, we tend to think of 'critical' as being a word with negative connotations when we use it in day-to-day discussion. When we use 'critical' in both an academic and a nursing environment, it has a more positive meaning. In clinical practice, the term 'critical' is concerned with risk, clinical awareness and precision. In academic work it relates to objectivity, judgement, reasoning and 'ruminative enquiry'. In academic work, an important aspect of being critical is to distinguish what is proven and defensible, and combine this with careful speculation.

ACTIVITY 3.1: HECTOR POPPY'S REFLECTION

Hector is writing a reflection for his portfolio. The focus of his reflection is his choice of wound care dressing for a patient with a leg ulcer. He knows that part of critical thinking is speculating, so he is speculating on the actions he could have taken.

(Continued)

I chose to use a simple non-adherent dressing to cover Mr B's leg ulcer, as, at the time, this seemed appropriate. However, on reviewing this decision, I now realise that there were other types of dressing I could have considered. Further investigation into this has identified that I could have used a silver-based dressing (Jemec et al., 2014), a honey dressing (Teobaldi and Motivari, 2018) or an alginate dressing (O'Meara et al., 2015).

Silver dressings are used to fight bacterial infections, a frequent problem with leg ulcers; honey dressings can help the ulcer heal, and alginate dressings are capable of absorbing large amounts of wound drainage. Thinking about this information, maybe any of these dressings would have been more appropriate for Mr B. He does have a bacterial infection in the wound, so perhaps the silver-based dressing would have helped to get rid of that. His wound is taking a very long time to heal; he has had it for three months now, so maybe the honey dressing would speed up the healing process. The alginate dressing might also have been a better idea than my simple non-adherent dressing, as his dressings are always very soggy when they are changed. An alginate dressing might absorb the exudate from Mr B's wound more effectively.

1. Does it seem surprising to you that speculation is part of critical thinking?
2. Can you see where the speculation is in Hector's reflection?
3. Read Hector's reflection again and think about what value speculating can bring.

Check the activity answers at the end of the chapter to see if our thoughts are similar.

Critical thinking is frequently viewed as a formal, refined and sophisticated activity, so it is possible that you may feel an activity such as speculating (which could also be thought of as wondering or guessing) should play no part. Speculating in critical thinking, however, enables you to imagine both what might be happening and what could be possible. Thus, speculation can assist to explain problems, help you to find solutions for them and identify strategies to explore other future possibilities.

This really is 'ruminative speculation', which involves developing theories that might explain the situation encountered (**inductive thinking**), and then applying and testing these theories (**deductive thinking**) (Rogal and Young, 2008). So, the sort of speculating we undertake in critical thinking isn't quite the same as wondering or guessing – it is a distant relative.

ANGUS'S REFLECTION AND SPECULATING

If we read Angus's reflection in Part A, we can see that he does some speculating in his 'So what?' section. He speculates: 'If I don't know enough, I might do the wrong thing. This could result in a patient not getting the right treatment.'

This is a good start and Angus is laying the foundation for critical thinking. He needs to do more than this, though, because even though he did engage in some speculation, he still needs to demonstrate his critical thinking more clearly. We will consider how he could do this later in the chapter, once we have developed our understanding of critical thinking further.

A (VERY) BRIEF HISTORY OF CRITICAL THINKING

Critical thinking is a **concept** that has been developed over the last 2,500 years, so there is a great deal of thought and writing on the topic.

The intellectual roots of critical thinking can be traced back to Socrates, who, 2,500 years ago, established the importance of asking questions that probe into the thinking behind ideas before they are accepted. Thus, it was Socrates who established the importance of seeking evidence, examining reasoning and assumptions, analysing ideas and thinking through the implications of what is being said or done.

Socrates' work was followed by the critical thinking of Plato and Aristotle, who both emphasised that things can often be very different from what they first appear to be. As a result of this, systematic critical thinking developed as a method to see through the way things look on the surface.

In the Middle Ages, thinkers such as Thomas Aquinas heightened awareness of the power of this method, and in the Renaissance, during the fifteenth and sixteenth centuries, many scholars in Europe began to think critically about art, religion, human nature and law. At this time, in England, a notable thinker, Francis Bacon, was particularly concerned about the way we 'misuse' our minds when we seek knowledge. He recognised that the mind cannot be left to 'natural thinking' and wrote an important book, *The Advancement of Learning*, which could be considered one of the earliest texts about critical thinking.

Over the following century, critical thinking was developed further by a number of thinkers, with Hobbes in particular outlining a naturalistic view of the world where everything was explained by evidence and reasoning. In the nineteenth century, this critical thought was extended further, leading to Darwin's *Descent of Men*.

From the twentieth century onwards, our understanding of the power of critical thinking has resulted in the recognition of the deep need for critical thinking in all aspects of life and education.

FINDING A DEFINITION OF CRITICAL THINKING

Due to the long history of critical thinking, it is unsurprising that there are numerous definitions of critical thinking, with several of these dating back many years. Figure 3.2 identifies some of the most frequently quoted definitions.

While these definitions are helpful and do provide some further understanding of what critical thinking is, they also raise many other questions that we need to answer.

From Figure 3.2, we can see that critical thinking relates to a range of intellectual skills that enable individuals to attain mastery of a specific subject. This level of mastery involves not just having expert knowledge, but also being able to apply evidence-based knowledge to new situations in order to come to sound conclusions. The use of evidence plays a very important role in critical thinking. In order to think critically, it is necessary to understand the importance of evidence and be able to both find relevant evidence and relate this to experience. As we have already said, in academic work an important aspect of being critical is to distinguish what is proven and defensible, and combine this with careful speculation. This is really what is meant in the feedback given to Faith, who we met at the start of the chapter. Using evidence to do this is fundamentally important, so we will consider further how evidence can be found and related to experience to achieve this later in this chapter.

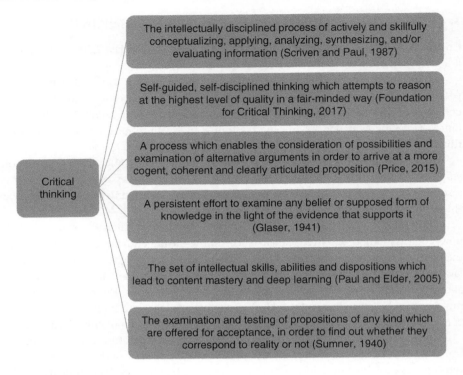

Figure 3.2   What is critical thinking?

As has been recognised by Socrates, Plato, Aristotle, Bacon, Darwin, and many other notable thinkers over the last 2,500 years, it is the use of evidence that makes critical thinking a very powerful tool. Table 3.1 outlines what we can gain by following the process of critical thinking.

Table 3.1   Critical thinking enables us to . . .

1. Consider a wide variety of viewpoints.

2. Analyse concepts, theories and explanations.

3. Clarify issues.

4. Examine assumptions.

5. Assess alleged facts.

6. Explore implications and consequences.

7. Think our way to conclusions.

8. Defend our thinking.

9. Solve problems.

10. Transfer ideas to new contexts.

11. Accept contradictions and inconsistencies in thoughts and experiences.

Source: Adapted from Paul and Elder (2005).

ACTIVITY 3.2

Review the 11 points identified in Table 3.1.

* How do you think each of these points could be helpful in your reflection?

Write down your thoughts and then compare them with mine in the answers at the end of the chapter.

THINKING CRITICALLY

As we can see from Table 3.1, if we are able to think critically, there is a wide variety of benefits to gain. One of the best ways to understand critical thinking is the examination and testing of **propositions** in order to find out whether they correspond to reality or not (Sumner, 1940). While this definition is over seventy years old, it still links very closely to what we do when we reflect. You may remember that in Chapter 1 we started our discussion about what reflection is with the very simple definition of reflection being 'thinking with a purpose'. Here is the link between critical thinking and reflection: a very important part of reflection is thinking and this needs to be critical. This will enable you to examine and test aspects of your experience and to question whether these aspects correspond with reality and thus provide effective patient care. As we have identified, this approach is called 'ruminative speculation', the developing of theories that might explain the situation encountered (inductive thinking), and then the application and testing of these theories (deductive thinking) (Rogal and Young, 2008). In order to think critically, however, just as highlighted by Faith at the start of the chapter, you need to be clear as to exactly what it is necessary to do. To understand this, we need to know a little more about the components of critical thinking.

Critical thinking has been described as being made up of two components – skills and commitment (Foundation for Critical Thinking, 2017) – as shown in Figure 3.3.

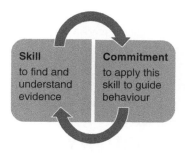

Skill to find and understand evidence   **Commitment** to apply this skill to guide behaviour

Figure 3.3   The two components of critical thinking

Source: Adapted from the Foundation for Critical Thinking (2017).

The first component of critical thinking is the skill to both find and process evidence. When considering this in respect of reflection, you will need to find evidence that relates to the aspect of the experience you are focusing on. Without having this evidence, you cannot begin to think critically about your experience.

The second component is the commitment to apply this skill to guide your behaviour. A good way to think of this second component is that you are using the evidence to indicate what is the most appropriate way for you to behave. It is this second component, the application of evidence, that identifies an individual as a critical thinker. A critical thinker's application of evidence to inform future behaviour marks them out as being very different from an individual who has memorised information or **learnt by rote**. The important difference is in the understanding of information. Traditionally, children in the UK were taught their times tables by rote and they would chant them in unison in order to commit them to memory. While this enabled children to quickly give the correct answer to the question, for example, 'What is 9 x 8?', such an approach did not provide them with a sound understanding of the principles of multiplication. Critical thinkers are very different. They constantly test, expand and apply their evidence-based knowledge and experience in order to adapt their behaviour. This also results in critical thinking becoming a skill that is constantly being developed. At the start of the chapter, Oscar wanted to know how he could become a more effective critical thinker. Table 3.2 identifies the features he needs to demonstrate.

Table 3.2   Features of a critical thinker

The ideal critical thinker is . . .	Critical thinkers are people . . .
• habitually inquisitive • well informed • trustful of reason • open-minded • honest in facing personal biases • prudent in making judgements • willing to reconsider • clear about issues • diligent in seeking relevant information • orderly in complex matters • reasonable in the selection of criteria • focused in enquiry • persistent in seeking results which are as precise as the subject and the circumstances of enquiry permit (after Facione, 1990)	• engaging in productive and positive activity • viewing their thinking as a process rather than an outcome • varying in their manifestations of critical thinking according to context • experiencing triggers to critical thinking as positive or negative • feeling comfortable with the emotive as well as the rationale elements of the critical thinking process (after Brookfield, 1987)

Source: Adapted from Jasper (2011), p. 69.

ACTIVITY 3.3

Review Table 3.2.

- How many of these features do you think you already possess?
- What evidence can you provide to support this view?

There is no definitive answer to this activity as the answer is personal to you, but it may be helpful to discuss your answer with your practice supervisor, a colleague or your university lecturer.

According to Elder (2006), critical thinking is self-guided, self-disciplined thinking which attempts to reason at the highest level of quality in a fair-minded way. This clearly is a very different approach from the immediate recall of isolated facts (or numbers).

Thinking is something we all do very naturally. We all think, all of the time. Left unrestrained, however, our thinking can become biased, distorted, uninformed and prejudiced. As we have already mentioned, this is where critical thinking differs from our everyday, **inherent** thinking. To think critically, we need to reason in a fair-minded way, so a **systematic** approach is required.

ACTIVITY 3.4

Find a recent written news report, either online, in a newspaper or on social media. Read the report and note any examples of:

fair-minded reasoning;

biased, distorted, uninformed or prejudiced reasoning.

- Having noted any examples, what conclusions can you come to about the quality of the news report?
- Bearing this in mind, would you say that within the news report there was evidence of effective critical thinking?

Write down your thoughts and then compare them with mine in the answers at the end of the chapter.

WHY DO I NEED TO THINK CRITICALLY WHEN REFLECTING?

As we have discussed, critical thinking requires the effort to examine any knowledge or belief in respect of the evidence that supports it in order to come to a sound conclusion. It also enables problems to be recognised and solved, plus any unsupported assumptions and values to be identified (Glaser, 1941). Critical thinking enables you to review your knowledge, beliefs and values in the light of wider experience and come to sound judgements. If we return to the start of Chapter 1 and review the definition of reflective practice – 'thinking about an experience and learning from it' – it seems that critical thinking and reflective practice are actually very tightly intertwined.

In order for your reflections to be effective, you need to ensure that you think critically while you are working through the stages of the reflective model you are applying. Critical thinking, just like reflection, is a process. Critical thinking in reflection tends to be an **introspective** activity that considers how values, attitudes, motives and skills relate to a particular context. As we already know, reflection considers the interactions of individuals and how they interpret an experience (Price and Harrington, 2013). So, in a reflection, for example, you might explore why you promoted a specific course of action to a patient. Going back to the question Oscar asked at the start of the chapter, to do this in an effective way that demonstrated critical thinking would involve reviewing:

- the evidence supporting the specific course of action;
- what your thoughts of the course of action are;
- what it is reasonable to expect the patient to do and why;
- why there might be areas of difficulty, either for the patient or for you.

Critical thinking in reflective practice involves a progressively deeper examination of meaning by exploring your personal values and beliefs, your rationale for understanding care in the way you do and how this influences the way you care for patients (Price and Harrington, 2013). As we said in Chapter 2, reflection really is all about you in that the objective is to learn more about yourself by considering your actions, knowledge, values, beliefs and feelings in respect of relevant evidence.

WHAT EVIDENCE AND WHERE FROM?

We have mentioned evidence frequently throughout this chapter so far, but haven't considered exactly what we actually mean by this. Evidence is both knowledge and information, and it is what we use to make decisions in all areas of our lives. Earlier in this chapter, we talked about using critical thinking skills in order to decide whether to have a big bar of chocolate or baked beans on toast for supper. Information (or evidence) was used in order to make a decision, evidence from experience in that you had eaten chocolate before and liked the taste, and evidence that identified the food with the best nutritional value.

When we are using information to support or question nursing practice, the evidence frequently comes from one or more of four sources (Thorpe and Delves-Yates, 2018).

ACTIVITY 3.5

- What do you think are the four different sources of evidence frequently used to support or question nursing practice?

Write down your thoughts and then compare them with mine in the answers at the end of the chapter.

While it is usually quite easy to find information about chocolate bars and baked beans because it is on the label, to find information (or evidence) about all aspects of nursing practice may not be so simple. The type of evidence we use most often to answer questions about nursing practice is theory or research evidence. However, it is possible that you may find that there may not be any theory or research evidence in existence to answer all your nursing questions. This could be either because your questions cannot be researched or because the research has not been undertaken yet. If this is the case, you would then need to use evidence from observation, reflection or patient experience to answer your question. In such situations, it is very important to be certain that the evidence you use is **trustworthy**, because you are using this evidence to make decisions about the nursing care you deliver to patients. Table 3.3 provides some guidance on how you can make a judgement as to the trustworthiness of evidence from your own nursing expertise.

Table 3.3   Is it trustworthy?

Evidence from	Issues to consider
Reflection and observation	• Is the context in which the care is being delivered similar?
	• Are there any professional, moral or ethical issues that need consideration?
	• Are there any clinical guidelines or manuals of nursing interventions that can provide further knowledge?
Patient experience	• What do patients value?
	• What do patients expect?

Source: Adapted from Thorpe and Delves-Yates, 2018, with kind permission of Gabrielle Thorpe.

Evidence from research is always viewed as providing the most reliable answers to questions. All research evidence is not thought of as being of the same value, however. Table 3.4 shows how research evidence is ranked in order of strength.

Table 3.4   Hierarchy of evidence

Type of evidence

Name	Description	Strongest
Systematic review of randomised controlled trials (RCT).	The combined results of a number of studies that use a very strict experimental design where there is random allocation of individuals to the treatment they will receive.	
Systematic review of non-randomised trials.	The combined results of a number of studies that use a very strict experimental design but individuals are not allocated to treatment by random methods.	
A randomised controlled trial (RCT).	The results of one study that uses a very strict experimental design where there is random allocation of individuals to the treatment they will receive.	
A non-randomised trial.	The results of one study that uses a very strict experimental design, but individuals are not allocated to treatment by random methods.	
Systematic reviews of correlational or observational studies.	The combined results of a number of studies that examine the links between causes and effects.	

(Continued)

Table 3.4   (Continued)

Type of evidence		
A correlational or observational study.	The results of one study that examines the links between causes and effects.	
Systematic reviews of descriptive or qualitative studies.	The combined results of a number of studies that describe an event or experience.	
A descriptive or qualitative study.	The results of one study that describes an event or experience.	
Opinions of authorities or expert committees.	The understanding and interpretations of a group of people who are experienced in a specific area.	**Weakest**

Source: Adapted from Thorpe and Delves-Yates, 2018, with kind permission of Gabrielle Thorpe.

Frequently in reflections, when we are considering feelings and experiences, the research evidence available to answer our questions will be at the lower end of the hierarchy of evidence. This really is not so surprising: drugs, for example, can be subjected to extensive scientific investigation, so it is relatively easy to conduct randomised control trials and systematic reviews of these. When we are considering feelings and experiences, randomised control trials and systematic reviews are much more difficult, if not impossible. This doesn't mean, however, that the knowledge from evidence at the lower end of the hierarchy of evidence isn't useful. You just need to remember that if you are using evidence from a study which explored the experience of one patient, it is not possible to apply this knowledge to every patient's experience without making sure it is trustworthy.

Once you have an understanding of the sort of evidence you want to find in order to support or question nursing practice in your reflection, the next step is to know where to find it. Table 3.5 offers some guidance.

Table 3.5   Where can I find it . . . ?

Where?	Positives	Negatives
The internet	Easy to access	Can be of poor quality.
	Lots of material	Lots of unofficial sites – are they trustworthy?
	Excellent 'official' sources of information and clinical guidelines such as:	Lots of the information available is aimed at patients – this might give you introductory information for the topic, but it is not going to be sufficiently detailed to support your nursing practice or academic work.
	• National Institute for Health and Care Excellence (NICE)	
	• Scottish Intercollegiate Guidelines Network (SIGN)	
	• Department of Health (DOH)	
	• Nursing and Midwifery Council (NMC)	
Databases of journal literature	Links to these are provided by universities and hospital libraries.	Can be of poor quality.
	Provides excellent evidence to support your nursing practice and academic work.	Lots of different databases – you need to know which one is most likely to provide you with the evidence you need.
		Need to know how to effectively search a database.

The best approach when looking for research evidence is to use a combination of both sources from the internet and databases. While searching databases effectively is a skill, it is one that either your hospital or university library will be able to assist you to master.

Before you can be sure that you have the evidence you require, there is just one final step to take. You cannot be certain of the quality of the evidence you find either on the internet or in a database of journal literature. Just because evidence has been published on the internet or in a journal, still does not mean that you can be certain that it is good evidence. You need to make a judgement about the literature and demonstrate in your reflection that you have done so. Referring back to Oscar's question at the start of the chapter, this is an important aspect of effective critical thinking. Judging evidence is a skill that takes time to develop, but there is help for you to do this. Seven simple questions you can ask yourself to help make this judgement are identified in Table 3.6.

Table 3.6   Judging quality

1. Does your evidence answer the question you were asking?

   If you have recently published evidence which is related to the topic you are considering but doesn't actually answer your question, it would be better to use an older piece of evidence, which precisely answers your question.

2. Who has published your evidence?

   If the evidence has been published in a high-quality, **peer-reviewed journal,** it is likely to be of better quality than evidence in a non-peer reviewed journal.

3. Who wrote your evidence?

   If your evidence is written by a key writer or researcher in the field, or it uses what you know to be key pieces of information to support the evidence it presents, it is likely to be of good quality.

4. Is the evidence supported by appropriate and varied sources of information?

   If there is a reference list containing what you know are the key pieces of information, it is more likely to be of good quality.

5. When was the evidence published?

   Apart from **seminal texts,** evidence should have been published within the past ten years.

6. Has the evidence been quoted by others?

   If the evidence has been cited in the reference list of other articles, for example, it will have been judged as high quality by others. (Some databases will enable you to check how many times an article has been cited.)

7. What is the view of a formal appraisal tool?

   There are many formal appraisal tools (such as the Critical Appraisal Skills Programme (CASP) tools) which can assist you to judge more fully the quality of primary research. This level of appraisal would not be expected for every piece of evidence, but if you have asked the previous six questions and are still uncertain as to the quality, undertaking a formal appraisal may enable you to make a confident judgement.

Source: Adapted from Thorpe and Delves-Yates, 2018, with kind permission of Gabrielle Thorpe.

Considering what has been written in this chapter so far, it may seem that you need to spend a great deal of time doing other things, such as finding and judging evidence, before you can start to write your reflection. That is true. If you want to produce a reflection that clearly demonstrates critical thinking, you are likely to find that the writing itself takes far

---

ACTIVITY 3.6

Find an article relating to a topic you are interested in, either by searching online or using an electronic library search engine. Read the article carefully and then answer the seven questions in Table 3.6.

- What is your judgement on the quality of the article?

There is no definitive answer to this activity, but you could discuss your view with a colleague, your practice supervisor or university lecturer.

---

less time than the thinking about it. In fact, to produce a written piece that demonstrates critical thinking takes a great deal of thinking. Here I am not talking about the 'distraction thinking' that can strike when you have a piece of work to produce, but can't really get down to it, so you start to think about summer holidays, what you are going to have for supper and all the other things you could be doing. The thinking we are talking about here is thinking about exactly what the focus of your reflection is and how you are going to write about it, thinking about whether you have all of the evidence you need, thinking about how the evidence relates to the questions you are asking and what that evidence actually tells you. Again, if like Oscar you want to make your critical thinking more effective, make sure that you don't start writing until you have done all this thinking. It is tempting to want to start writing before you have done all the preparation. If you do this, you are very likely to find that you will get stuck because you haven't thought enough to have anything to write about.

HOW DO I WRITE IN A WAY THAT DEMONSTRATES CRITICAL THINKING?

As we have said, writing is hard work, but as it is a skill that will improve with practice, this is hard work you need to do. As you refine what you are writing, it will assist your thinking,

> *structuring and restructuring, seeking explanations and new ways of knowing, leads us to look for unique explanations in themselves that may direct action and affect outcomes for our clients*

> Jasper (2011, p. 71)

So, the process of writing is an important aspect of critical thinking which will help you to develop your thoughts.

Table 3.7 has a number of tips to help you get started and practise writing in a way that demonstrates critical thinking. You may remember a very similar table in Chapter 2, Table 2.1, which showed you how Borton's (1970) model could be used to write a reflection. Table 3.7 develops this by providing prompts for the questions you need to answer and information you need to include in order to make your reflection critical. If we go back to the questions asked by Faith and Oscar at the start of the chapter, the hints and tips in Table 3.7 will help them, and you, to demonstrate critical thinking in your writing.

Table 3.7 Critical thinking tips

Borton's (1970) model of reflection: What?, So what?, What now?	Reflection tips	Critical thinking tips
What? Essential elements included in this stage: • critical incident; • description. This is the description of your critical incident. Here you write an overview of your experience describing: • What was the context for the experience? • Why is this experience important to you? • What happened? • How you were involved? • What exactly did you do? • What were your thoughts and feelings? • How did you respond to what happened?	Focus on just one aspect of your experience so you can consider this issue in detail, rather than trying to consider lots of issues and not achieving any depth in your reflection. Make sure that your description is clear, so that the reader fully understands your experience. You are unlikely to be able to write a clear description on the first attempt at writing down your experience, so keep reading what you have written and refine it, until it says exactly what you want it to. At this point it can be useful to ask a friend to read what you have written and give you some feedback.	To get your reflection off to a good start: 1. ensure that you are not overly ambitious in what you chose to cover – less really is more, as then you will be able to discuss issues in detail; 2. clearly identify what you are aiming to achieve. Jasper et al. (2013) suggest reflecting using SODA, which stands for **S**ignificance, **O**utcome, **D**escribable, **A**ction. While this can be used as a model in itself, if it is used in conjunction with other prompt questions, it can be useful in assisting critical thinking. The S, O and D part of SODA can be helpful for your critical thinking in this stage of Borton's (1970) model. **Significance:** Why was it significant? Why does it stand out in your mind? What is important about this incident? **Outcome:** What do you want to achieve as a result of this experience? What might you learn from it to help your practice? What might you learn about yourself?

(Continued)

Table 3.7 (Continued)

Borton's (1970) model of reflection: What?, So what?, What now?

Reflection tips	Critical thinking tips
	Describable:
	How can you describe it?
	What are the constraints?
	What may be the consequences?
	What are the ethical issues?
	What are the professional implications?
So what?	This stage of the model has lots of opportunities to demonstrate critical thinking. Make sure that you use relevant evidence to support your writing so it is very clear how you know what you are stating. Get in to the habit of supporting all the statements you make with evidence.
Essential elements included in this stage:	
• analysis;	
• interpretation;	3. Identify and challenge any assumptions you made – this could relate to, for example, knowledge, values, actions, beliefs, emotions, the role of the patient, the role of the nurse, power, political issues, economic circumstances, decisions, etc.
• perspective.	
This is where you break the experience down so you can question:	
• What was important in this experience?	4. What is actually happening in your experience?
	5. Is anything important missing?
• What were your thoughts and feelings during the experience?	6. What are the influences?
	7. What if?
• What theory relates to your experience?	8. What was the aim of your actions?
• What went well?	9. What were your reasons for undertaking your actions?
• What could have gone better?	10. Does the evidence support your reasons?
• What were the consequences of your actions and beliefs?	11. What are the assumptions behind your reasons?
	12. What does all of this mean?
• Does the experience make you rethink your actions and beliefs?	13. Have you considered all of the who, what, where, when, why, how?
• What did the experience teach you?	As mentioned in the previous section, Jasper et al. (2013) suggest we can reflect using SODA. In this section we could again consider the O and D of the model by discussing the following issues, but rather than repeating any previous discussion, develop this further.
• How do your personal and professional values relate to the experience?	

In this stage the aim is to clearly demonstrate that you have carefully considered your experience and thought about the relationship between theoretical principles and practice.

Your consideration needs to include discussion relating to the consequences of your actions and beliefs, and if relevant those of any others involved.

You need to provide evidence that you are aware of both your personal and professional values.

To produce an effective reflection which achieves Goodman's Level 2 or 3, this section needs to use references to support the statements you are making. This will enable you to identify the reasoning behind and the evidence base of the actions you took.

Borton's (1970) model of reflection: What?, So what?, What now?	Reflection tips	Critical thinking tips
• What would you do differently if you were faced with a similar situation – what would be the different actions or approaches you could take? • What is the significance of what happened? • What else do you need to consider to understand more fully what happened? • What sense can you make of this experience? • How did this experience influence or change you?	To achieve Goodman's Level 3, you also need to consider the broader social structures and forces, plus the wider influences of ethical and political decisions with regard to care delivery and practice.	Outcome: What did you achieve as a result of the experience? What did you learn from the experience to help your practice? What did you learn about yourself? Describable: How did you deal with the consequences of your actions? How did you deal with the ethical issues? How will the professional issues influence your future practice?
What now? Essential element included in this stage: action. This is where you put things back together – the synthesis – and relate this experience to your future considering: • What do you need to do now? • What do I need to learn following my experience? • How are you going to do this?	It is important in this section to demonstrate that you understand the need to know more and the actions you are going to take to achieve this.	In this section you need to show that you have thought critically about what you can improve and/or how you will act differently as a result of your experience. Again, using the evidence to show how you have considered this will demonstrate your critical thinking. Remember that you need to be: 14. objective, so while there may be some parts of your actions you want to improve upon, there will also be some parts of your actions that went well; 15. honest about your thoughts, as this will enable you to both learn from your experience and learn about yourself. Again, we can use SODA (Jasper et al., 2013). In this section we could again consider the A of the model by discussing the following issues: Action: What actions do you need to take? Who else can help you?

As you can see from Table 3.7, there is a great deal to consider when you are writing a reflection. Critical thinking is fundamentally important in aiding you to learn from your experiences, as critical thinking and reflective practice are very tightly intertwined. An important aspect of critical thinking is being systematic – applying the critical tips identified in Table 3.7 will help you to think in a logical manner. However, the best way to develop your ability to both reflect and think critically is to practise. The more you write in a reflective and critical way about your experiences, the better you will get at it. Chapter 4 provides further guidance as to how you can improve your ability to write in a reflexive manner, so make time to read this as well as practising reflecting.

ACTIVITY 3.7

Using your literature searching skills, find the article written by Duffy, K., Hastie, E., McCallum, J., Ness, V. and Price, V. (2009) Academic writing: using literature to demonstrate critical analysis, *Nursing Standard*, 23(47): 35-40. While this article is over ten years old and contains some information about nurse education which is now dated, the information it provides relating to how to use evidence to demonstrate critical thinking is excellent. From that perspective, it therefore remains valid.

   Read the article and, based on the numerous tips it outlines, add your own tips to Table 3.7 in order to provide personal prompts that will assist you to demonstrate critical thinking in your reflection.

There is no definitive answer for this activity, as all answers will be individual.

HOW DOES ANGUS DEMONSTRATE CRITICAL THINKING IN HIS REFLECTION?

If we read Angus's reflection in Part A, we can see that he makes reference to *The Code* (NMC, 2018), which is a good attempt at supporting his statements about not knowing enough and ensuring that patients are given good care with evidence. If we look at Table 3.7, though, and read through the Critical thinking tips column, we can see that there are many questions that Angus could consider in the So what? section. It seems as if he is thinking about the assumption he made, that he should know what to do on his first day, but he needed to give us more details so that we could be certain this was what he was saying, and then use evidence to challenge his assumption. Angus mentions his experience when he was a volunteer teacher and how his feelings were similar, but exactly what he means isn't clear. It seems as if he is trying to challenge the assumption that he should know what to do by mentioning his first day as a volunteer teacher, but Angus hasn't actually said this, so we are interpreting what he means. Angus needs to work more on his reflection to make what he means clearer. He needs to be more explicit about what he assumed and use more evidence to clearly challenge this assumption. Angus then needs to make a judgement as to whether his assumption was valid, clearly saying whether he was correct to think he should know what to do on his first day on placement or whether this is not achievable. Again, he has gone some way to do this, but has not made his thinking in this section sufficiently clear.

However, Angus has done a very good job in the What now? section. If you compare what he has written with the Critical thinking tips column from Table 3.7, he has achieved the points identified.

So, Angus has made a good start with his first reflection, but he can make it even better. To do this, Angus will need to keep working on the reflection, reviewing and refining the sections to ensure that exactly what he is thinking about is clear. He can also learn from the other nurses he meets on his placement to find out how they use critical thinking and to see how he can apply what they do to his practice.

CONCLUSION

Critical thinking is a concept that has been developed over the last 2,500 years and which is now part of all aspects of life and education, as it brings many benefits.

There is a strong link between critical thinking and reflection. Applying critical thinking when we reflect enables us to examine and test aspects of our experience. This enables us to question whether our experience corresponds with reality and thus provides effective patient care.

What is meant by the term 'critical thinking' may at first seem confusing. What we need to do, however, is to be objective, think about a topic in great detail, ask questions, consider the evidence and finally arrive at a logical conclusion. While this might seem daunting, just like riding a bicycle, critical thinking is a skill. So, with hard work and practice, your critical thinking ability will improve.

--------------------- GOING FURTHER ---------------------

Delves-Yates, C. (ed.) (2018) *Essentials of Nursing Practice* (2nd edn). London: SAGE. Chapters 3 and 4 are excellent and will help you to understand both the importance of evidence and how you find and use it.

Price, B. (2015) Applying critical thinking to nursing. *Nursing Standard*, 29(51): 49–58. This excellent article aims to provide a clear understanding of the different types and levels of critical thinking that relate to both theoretical and reflective forms of writing.

Can critical thinking skills be taught? Go to: www.youtube.com/watch?v=BHGurFcEShw. An interesting video considering this topic and providing hints to improve your critical thinking in nursing.

--------------------- ANSWERS TO ACTIVITIES ---------------------

Activity 3.1

1. Hector is writing a reflection for his portfolio. The focus of his reflection is his choice of wound care dressing for a patient with a leg ulcer. He knows that part of critical thinking is speculating, so he is speculating on the actions he could have taken.

(Continued)

... I chose to use a simple non-adherent dressing to cover Mr B's leg ulcer as, at the time, this seemed appropriate. However, on reviewing this decision, I now realise that there were other types of dressing I could have considered. Further investigation into this has identified that I could have used a silver-based dressing (Jemec et al., 2014), a honey dressing (Teobaldi and Motivari, 2018) or an alginate dressing (O'Meara et al., 2015).

Silver dressings are used to fight bacterial infections, a frequent problem with leg ulcers, honey dressings can help the ulcer heal and alginate dressings are capable of absorbing large amounts of wound drainage. Thinking about this information, ...

2.   Hector is speculating here ...

maybe any of these dressings would have been more appropriate for Mr B. He does have a bacterial infection in the wound, so perhaps the silver-based dressing would have helped to get rid of that. His wound is taking a very long time to heal – he has had it for three months now, so maybe the honey dressing would speed up the healing process. The alginate dressing might also have been a better idea than my simple nonadherent dressing, as his dressings are always very soggy when they are changed. An alginate dressing might absorb the exudate from Mr B's wound more effectively.

3.   The speculation Hector is undertaking is not the same as guessing; he is using new knowledge of wound dressings to think about what might be possible. So, his speculation in this reflection is very valuable, as it is helping him to understand how the care given to Mr B might be improved. This speculation is going to help Hector to find a dressing which has been specifically designed to help with the healing of Mr B's wound. So, by speculating Hector is developing his understanding of what might be possible in the care of Mr B's wound, and identifying a more effective wound dressing than the one currently being used.

Activity 3.2

1.   Considering a wide variety of viewpoints ensures that your reflection is well informed.
2.   Analysing concepts, theories and explanations ensures that your reflection is based on relevant and appropriate evidence.
3.   Clarifying issues ensures that the reader understands exactly what you are discussing.
4.   Examining assumptions ensures that the conclusions you have made are based on sound evidence, not individual views.
5.   Assessing alleged facts ensures that your writing is based on sound evidence.
6.   Exploring implications and consequences ensures that you have carefully considered all potential outcomes of any conclusions you have made.
7.   Thinking your way to conclusions ensures that the conclusions you have come to are logical and appropriate.
8.   Defending your thinking, ensuring you are able to quote the evidence it is based on, provides certainty that your thoughts are logical and appropriate.
9.   Solving problems, ensuring you apply the relevant evidence to guide your actions.
10. Transferring ideas to new contexts, ensuring the sharing and development of evidence-based practice.
11. Accepting contradictions and inconsistencies in thoughts and experiences, ensuring that you always recognise that just as all patients and nurses are unique, so are the experiences they create.

Activity 3.4

1. While each news report will be different, any examples of biased, distorted, uninformed or prejudiced reasoning would make it difficult to have any confidence that the news being reported was from an objective perspective. This would make the quality of the news report poor.

2. Evidence of critical thinking would be demonstrated by the inclusion of the following:

    a. Clear identification of:

        1. the key ideas, problems, arguments, observations, findings, conclusions;
        2. evidence to support the problems, arguments, observations, findings, conclusions;
        3. a writing style that distinguishes fact from opinion and outlines any bias.

    b. Evaluation of:

        • the evidence;
        • any assumptions being made.

    c. A consistent and logical line of reasoning.
    d. Use of unemotive and unbiased language.

Activity 3.5

The four sources of evidence frequently used are:

• observation;
• reflection;
• patient experience;
• theory/research.

GLOSSARY

concept   An idea, notion or thought.

deductive thinking   Reasoning that starts with a general theory or statement and works its way to an evidence-based conclusion.

inductive thinking   Reasoning that starts with an observation or questions and works its way to a theory by examining the relevant evidence.

inherent   In-built.

introspective   Inward-looking.

learnt by rote   A memorisation technique based on repetition.

objective   Not influenced by personal feelings or interpretations.

peer-reviewed journal   An academic publication where articles are reviewed by several other experts in the field before they are published. Thus the articles are more likely to be of good quality.

propositions   Proposals, suggestions or intentions.

seminal texts   Highly influential information written on a particular topic which is frequently cited.

systematic   Applying a comprehensive, methodical and logical approach.

trustworthy   Dependable, reliable and honest.

REFERENCES

Borton, T. (1970) *Reach, Touch and Teach*. London: Hutchinson.

Brookfield, S.D. (1987) *Developing Critical Thinkers: Challenging Adults to Explore Alternative Ways of Thinking and Acting*. San Francisco, CA: Jossey Bass.

Elder, L. (2006) *The Miniature Guide to Critical Thinking for Children*. Dillon Beach, CA: Foundation for Critical Thinking.

Facione, PA (1990) *The Delphi Report. Critical Thinking: A Statement of Export Consensus for Purposes of Educational Assessment and Instruction*. Executive Summary. Berkeley, CA: The California Academic Press.

Foundation for Critical Thinking (2017) Another brief conceptualization of critical thinking. Available at: www.criticalthinking.org/pages/defining-critical-thinking/766 (accessed 22 August 2020).

Glaser, E.M. (1941) *An Experiment in the Development of Critical Thinking*. Teacher's College, Columbia University.

Jasper, M. (2011) Understanding reflective writing. In Rolfe, G., Jasper, M. and Freshwater, D. *Critical Reflection in Practice* (2nd edn). Basingstoke: Palgrave Macmillan.

Jasper, M., Rosser, M. and Mooney, G. (2013) *Professional Development, Reflection and Decision Making in Nursing and Health Care* (2nd edn). Chichester: John Wiley & Sons.

Nursing and Midwifery Council (NMC) (2018) *The Code*. London: NMC.

Jemec, G.B.E., Kerihuel, J.C., Ousey, K., Lauemøller, S.L. and Leaper, D.J. (2014) Cost-effective use of silver dressings for the treatment of hard-to-heal chronic venous leg ulcers. *PLoS ONE, 9*(6): e100582. Available at: https://doi.org/10.1371/journal.pone.0100582

O'Meara, S., Martyn-St James, M. and Adderley, U.J. (2015) Alginate dressings for venous leg ulcers. *Cochrane Database of Systematic Reviews*, 8. Art. No.: CD010182. DOI: 10.1002/14651858.CD010182.pub3.

Paul, R. and Elder, L. (2005) *Critical Thinking Competency Standards*. Dillon Beach, CA: Foundation for Critical Thinking.

Price, B. and Harrington, A. (2013) *Critical Thinking and Writing for Nursing Students* (2nd edn). London: SAGE.

Price, B. (2015) Applying critical thinking to nursing. *Nursing Standard, 29*(51): 49–58.

Rogal, S.M. and Young, J. (2008) Exploring critical thinking in critical care nursing education: a pilot study. *Journal of Continuing Education in Nursing, 39*(1): 28–33.

Scriven, M. and Paul, R. (1987) Defining Critical Thinking. 8th Annual International Conference on Critical Thinking and Education Reform. Available at: www.criticalthinking.org/pages/defining-critical-thinking/766 (accessed 21 October 2020).

Sumner, W.G. (1940) *Folkways: A Study of the Sociological Importance of Usages, Manners, Customs, Mores, and Morals*. New York: Ginn & Co.

Teobaldi, I. and Montivari, A. (2018) Pressure heel ulcers in patients with type 2 diabetes: Is it T.I.M.E. to customise wound bed preparation according to different heel areas? *International Wound Journal, 15*: 849–50.

Thorpe, G. and Delves-Yates, C. (2018) Core Academic Skills. In Delves-Yates, C. (ed.) *Essentials of Nursing Practice* (2nd edn). London: SAGE.

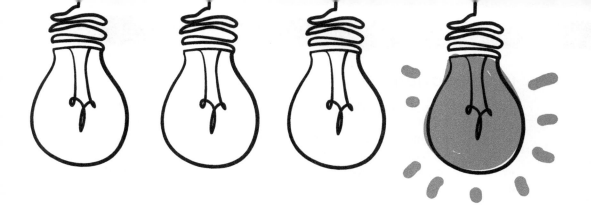

WRITING REFLECTIVELY

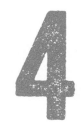

4

CATHERINE DELVES-YATES

I am trying to write a reflection for my revalidation, but . . . ! Can I write in the first person in work that is for a formal purpose? Will it sound like I am writing a letter to a friend rather than an academic piece? If I don't say 'I, me and my', though, what do I say – the author, the reflector? That doesn't sound right!

John Angelinetta, registered nurse, learning disability field

The feedback about my last reflection said that I included too much description and not enough reflection. I am really not sure about the difference between them. The reflective model I used said to describe my experience, so I did. Now I am confused – what should I do?

Victoria Curtis, nursing student, adult field

INTRODUCTION

As John tells us at the very start of the chapter, reflective writing is an important aspect of reflection for formal purposes, but, as we will discuss later in the chapter, it can also be part of informal, much more personal reflections, such as reflective diaries. Writing reflectively can seem rather a challenge, especially as it is likely to be a very different writing style to the one usually associated with formal writing. It isn't, however, quite as difficult as it might seem at first, and with a clear understanding of what you are aiming to achieve plus plenty of practice, it is a skill that you can both master and enjoy.

In this chapter we are going to consider exactly what reflective writing is and why we need to undertake it. We will build on the steps we have taken in the previous chapters, consider hints and tips to help you write reflectively plus review Angus's reflection in Part A, to show how it could be improved. Following the process of improving Angus's reflection will help you understand what strategies you can apply to your reflective writing in order to improve it.

──────────── CHAPTER AIMS ────────────

This chapter will enable you to:

- understand what is meant by reflective writing;
- appreciate why we need to write reflectively;
- recognise the importance of reflective thinking;
- clearly demonstrate effective reflective writing in your own reflections.

WHAT IS REFLECTIVE WRITING?

Reflective writing is a written account that analyses and examines an experience. The aim of reflective writing is to consider the meaning and impact of the experience, and the process of writing reflectively provides the writer with insights of their experience which leads to learning about themselves. Thus, reflective writing can be thought of as the rewinding of experience and the thinking of how it affected you, what you could have done differently to change the outcome and what the result was. When you produce a piece of reflective writing you will have your own personal interpretation of the experience that identifies what it means to you, what you have learned and how you can apply this learning in the future. As we have said in previous chapters, reflection is all about you, and therefore, so is reflective writing.

WHY DO WE NEED TO WRITE REFLECTIVELY?

Reflective writing is frequently used as a way to demonstrate the ability to think reflectively. While this is often for a formal purpose, to demonstrate careful consideration of an experience for revalidation, for example, as is the case with John who we met at the start of the chapter, using reflective writing in a more personal manner is also highly valuable, as it is an excellent way to learn about your thoughts and feelings. A reflective diary is a good example of using reflective writing in a more personal manner, as is shown in Figure 4.1.

> 12th November 2020
>
> Today I had to give a presentation on fractures. This has been the most challenging part of the course for me so far, as it isn't something I have done before. I was so very nervous to start with, my words all got in a bit of a jumble!! However, because I had written notes and practised what I was going to say, I got over this and finished.
>
> I can't say I enjoyed doing it, but I am very pleased that I did, and I don't think I made too bad a job. I got a big round of applause from the other students, who even said it was good!
>
> What I have learned is when I have to do it again I must be prepared and practise. Well, actually I think being prepared and practising is a good plan for lots of things, not just for giving a presentation.

Figure 4.1 A reflective diary entry

Taking ten minutes at the end of each day to write briefly in a reflective manner about an experience that happened during the day is an excellent way to practise your reflective writing. Keeping a reflective diary will also help you to carefully consider your personal feelings about, for example, learning something new, or overcoming a barrier, or maybe a 'lightbulb moment' when something you had been puzzling over for a while became clear.

ACTIVITY 4.1

Set yourself the target of keeping a reflective diary for the next two weeks. Spend ten minutes each day writing about something you think is important that happened during the day. While this writing is purely for you, in order for it to help you develop your reflective writing skills, make sure that you:

(Continued)

- write in full sentences, not just notes;
- check your spelling and grammar;
- maintain confidentiality.

Getting into the habit of keeping a reflective diary will ensure that your ten minutes of 'personal writing' each day also develops your ability to write in a professional manner. If you find it difficult to get started with your writing, think about how you would answer the question, 'What have I learned about myself today?' and use the 'free writing' approach we discussed in Chapter 2.

When you have written your diary each day for two weeks, take time to reread the entries you have written and answer the following questions:

1.   How has my reflective writing improved over the last two weeks?
2.   What has keeping a reflective diary helped me to realise about myself?

There is no definitive answer for this activity as it is based on your own experience, but you could discuss what you have found out with your practice supervisor, a colleague or university lecturer.

Gibbs (1988), who developed a reflective cycle you may have already used or, if not, will meet in Chapter 10, identified the importance of thinking about experience:

> *It is not sufficient to have an experience in order to learn. Without reflecting on the experience it may quickly be forgotten, or its learning potential lost*

> Gibbs (1988, p. 9)

Taking Gibbs's thoughts one step further, one of the best ways to ensure that an experience and the learning it resulted in are not forgotten is to keep a written record of it. Thus, reflective writing is a fundamentally important aspect in your development, either as a nursing student or registered nurse.

REFLECTIVE WRITING

As we have said, reflective writing is all about you. As shown in Figure 4.2, it is easy to think of reflection as looking in a mirror, in order to inspect yourself.

What is shown in Figure 4.2, however, isn't actually quite sufficient. To get to know yourself fully, you need to consider yourself from all angles, not just from the front. So, you would need to be completely surrounded by mirrors in order to see yourself in 360 degrees. Some of you might find this idea exciting, but others might find it rather scary. Even if we did stand in the middle of so many mirrors, though, there is still a problem. When we look in a mirror, we only see our physical body – what is on the outside. Reflection is concerned with what is on your inside – the thoughts, feelings, beliefs, values that make you the unique individual you are. Thus, reflective writing is much better than a mirror for revealing this to us. Writing reflectively on a regular basis is a

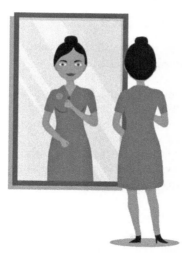

Figure 4.2   Reflection

very effective way of gaining a clear view of and understanding the thoughts, feelings, beliefs, values you hold. Once you have this knowledge about your 'inside', you can use it to develop yourself further.

When we talk about the view we have of ourselves in this way, we are actually talking about self-awareness. For nurses, being self-aware is very important, as having knowledge about yourself will help you to develop effective therapeutic relationships with patients.

Self-awareness is best described as the process of examining yourself objectively, which is not an easy task. Being self-aware takes time to achieve and may be a painful process, as you may realise things about yourself you don't like. It is also a process that is never quite finished; for as long as you live you will have new experiences and, following these experiences, your thoughts, feelings, beliefs and values may alter. We never stop learning about ourselves.

The term **introspection** is frequently mentioned when self-awareness is being considered. Introspection is when you **cognitively** explore, or think deliberately and carefully about your own thoughts, feelings, beliefs, values, behaviours and the feedback you receive from others. This is an important point to remember. When we reflect, we often focus on an experience, but, as we have said in previous chapters, trying to reflect on a whole experience makes it impossible to discuss everything that happened in depth. So, and this is especially important if we have only ten minutes to do some reflective writing, it is necessary to be very focused on the topic we reflect on. We might decide to focus on the actions we undertook in an experience – for example, how we performed the actions involved in dressing a wound. Such a reflection could be very useful, but if we want to learn about ourselves it could be even more useful to consider:

- our thoughts during an experience;
- our feelings during an experience;
- what we believe following an experience;
- what values an experience has enabled us to realise that we hold;
- any constructive criticism we have been given.

CONSTRUCTIVE CRITICISM

Constructive criticism, or what is often called feedback, is frequently given to us.
Formal feedback comes in two forms:

1. A planned and systematic part of the marking of any assessment, written or practical. This feedback will be written and given to you in respect of your ability to achieve the standard required to pass the assessment, highlighting what you did well and what you need to improve on.
2. The thoughts on your performance from others who are also involved in the activity. This is usually given verbally – for example, when you ask a patient for feedback on the care you are giving.

Formal feedback is a very useful source of information, but we need either to be undertaking an assessment or actively asking those around us to provide it. If we are observant, however, we can gain informal feedback on just about every action we undertake.

Informal feedback is freely available, if we look for it. For example, have you ever been sitting next to someone who says something you think is incorrect? How did you respond to this? You may have questioned them about their statement, or you may just have raised an eyebrow in a questioning fashion. These are both examples of informal feedback, and non-verbal informal feedback in particular is important to look out for because it is always available. As shown in the example of the raising of an eyebrow to show questioning of what was said, if we are observant, it is possible to receive feedback relating to our actions and care-giving without asking for it. Next time you are caring for a patient, as well as asking them for formal feedback on the care they are receiving, watch their body language to pick up on the non-verbal informal feedback they are giving you. It is an important part of your role as a nurse to interpret and act on it.

While feedback of any type is useful and will provide an excellent focus for a reflection, informal feedback is particularly valuable. This allows you to respond to, for example, a change in a patient's body language, showing how they are feeling without giving you formal, spoken feedback.

THE REFLECT-WELL PLATE

If we want to stay healthy, we all know how important it is to eat a varied diet. While having cake for every meal might, at first, sound good, it would eventually become boring and would definitely not be nutritious. It is much better to include some of all of the elements that make up the eat-well plate (PHE, 2016) if we want our diet to be healthy. We can think about reflection in the same way. While we frequently talk about reflection on an experience, doing only this can be rather like constantly eating cake. Unless we have the time, motivation and, if we are reflecting for an assessment, the word allowance, always focusing on an entire experience doesn't provide us with a sound balance. Taking a more balanced approach and sometimes making our thoughts, feelings, beliefs, values or feedback the focus of a reflection provides a much more effective approach. In this way, we can consider and start to understand, in detail, how our thoughts, feelings, beliefs, values and feedback motivate our actions. Think of what you choose to reflect on in the same way as you do the eat-well plate (PHE, 2016) in your diet, as shown in Figure 4.3, and remember that 'a little bit of everything does you good'.

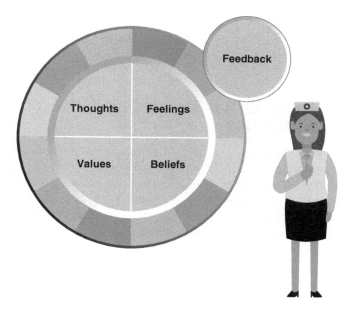

Figure 4.3   The reflect-well plate

REFLECTIVE THINKING

While the focus of this chapter is the act of reflective writing, the most important part of reflective writing is actually the thinking behind it. Reflective writing is the proof of reflective thinking, which is important because it is the link between experience and learning. A good piece of reflective writing clearly demonstrates to the reader that you have carefully considered the experience in a reflective fashion. If you are submitting your reflective writing for a formal purpose, it is the reflective thinking behind it that will gain you more marks than your ability to produce good reflective writing alone. As we have discussed in previous chapters, there are many ways to define reflection, and one that is particularly helpful when considering reflective thinking is that reflection is the art of looking backwards in order to see how you can apply the learning from your experience to the future (Shankar-Kay, 2016). When you reflect, you actually need to look both backwards and forwards. The ability to look both forwards into the future and backwards into the past is known as the Janus effect (see Figure 4.4) after Janus, a Roman god, who was able to look forwards and backwards with equal clarity.

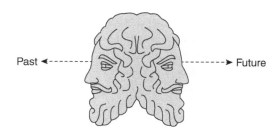

Figure 4.4   The Janus effect

Remember Janus when you are writing reflectively and ensure that you include the application of what has happened in the past (looking backwards) to what you plan for the future (looking forwards).

HOW CAN I PRODUCE A GOOD PIECE OF REFLECTIVE WRITING?

Although having the ability to 'write well' is advantageous, it is actually the content of your reflective writing that is of the utmost significance. So, as well as remembering Janus, when writing for a formal purpose, make sure that you include all the important elements we identified in Chapter 3, especially Table 3.7, to ensure that the content of your reflection is correct. Think of this as your recipe for producing the best reflection you can and, just like baking a cake, make sure that you always include all the ingredients, as otherwise, in the same way that if you forget to put the sultanas in a fruitcake, the end result won't be as good as you would like it to be.

ACTIVITY 4.2

Refer to Table 3.7 in Chapter 3 which provides you with the 'recipe' for a reflection. Throughout the rest of this chapter, we are going to make some final additions to this table, so in preparation for this, read all the columns to refamiliarise yourself and make a note of further personal hints and tips you think will be helpful.

There is no definitive answer for this activity.

In addition to ensuring that you include all the important aspects of reflection we have discussed up to now in your reflective writing, there are a few further elements to add. We identified Table 3.7 in Chapter 3 as our recipe for reflection; if this recipe had produced a cake, what we are going to do now is add the icing to it.

FORMALLY INFORMAL

At the start of this chapter, John was trying to work out the correct 'voice' to use when writing reflectively. He was unsure whether he should be saying 'I, me and my' and, if he did, how he could stop his writing feeling as if it was a letter to a friend. John is exactly right to want to use the first person (I, me and my) when writing his reflection. As we have mentioned previously, reflection is all about you, so 'I, me and my' are exactly the correct **personal pronouns** to use. If we look at a section of Angus's reflection (see Figure 4.5), this is what he does.

In his reflection, Angus has the **tone** of his writing exactly right and he sounds knowledgeable and accurate. He uses 'I, me and my' to relate all the discussion back to

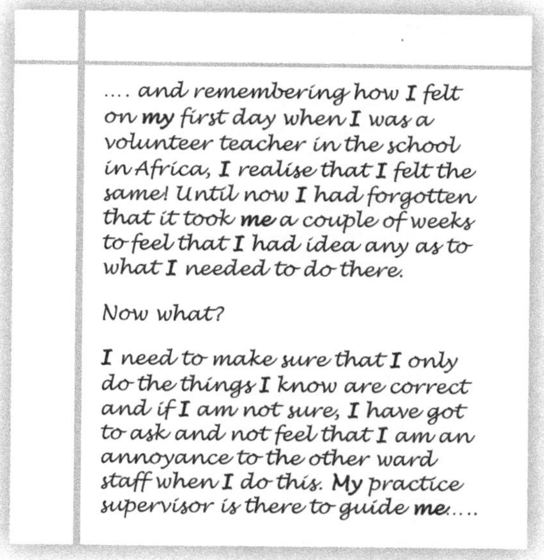

.... *and remembering how I felt on my first day when I was a volunteer teacher in the school in Africa, I realise that I felt the same! Until now I had forgotten that it took me a couple of weeks to feel that I had idea any as to what I needed to do there.*

Now what?

I need to make sure that I only do the things I know are correct and if I am not sure, I have got to ask and not feel that I am an annoyance to the other ward staff when I do this. My practice supervisor is there to guide me.....

Figure 4.5   I, me and my

ACTIVITY 4.3

Count the number of times Angus uses 'I, me and my' in the extract from his reflection in Figure 4.5. Does what he has written sound like a letter, something John was concerned about at the start of the chapter?

Check the activity answers at the end of the chapter to see if we agree.

---

himself and his experience. As we have said, when you have produced a piece of reflective writing, you will have your own personal interpretation of the experience which identifies what it means to you, what you have learned and how you can apply this learning in the future. Reflection is all about you, and reflective writing is writing to learn about yourself. Because of this personal element, reflective writing is written in a different way to, for example, a critical discussion or a literature review. One of the features of reflective writing is its specific style. This can be thought of as being formally informal, with the informality coming from the use of the personal pronouns 'I, me and my'. It is important to ensure that the academic tone of reflective writing is personal, but not 'chatty'. Reflective writing must not be too informal or it is in danger of becoming more like a letter to a friend. The way to ensure that you have the correct academic tone in your reflection is to use relevant evidence to analyse your experience, which will prevent your writing from being 'chatty' and **anecdotal**. There are further important features of reflective writing (see Table 4.1) that we also need to remember to include, as these will help to ensure that your reflective writing does not sound too informal.

Table 4.1 Important features of reflective writing

Reflective writing . . .

is written in a personal manner – is formally informal

- use personal pronouns such as 'I, me and my'

investigates an experience in a focused manner

- consider only one or two topics, as otherwise you will not be able to discuss them in sufficient depth

critically analyses what has happened

- use relevant literature to discuss and explain the situation, linking your experience to theory

highlights implications for the future

- include an action plan at the end to show how you will apply what you have learned to your future practice

REFLECTION AND DESCRIPTION

At the start of the chapter we met Victoria who was puzzling over the difference between reflection and description in order to understand how much description she should include in her reflection. Victoria is right to question this, as when there is too much description, the writing will be a purely descriptive account of her experience, otherwise known as a story. Victoria's dilemma is very common, because it is much easier to write descriptively than to stretch your brain and think reflectively. As we have already discussed, however, it is the reflective thinking that is most important, so we need to ensure that our reflective writing demonstrates this clearly. The difference between reflection and description is shown in Figure 4.6.

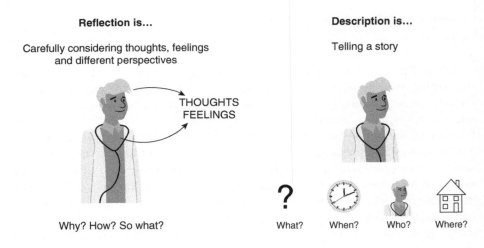

Reflection is...	**Description is...**
Carefully considering thoughts, feelings and different perspectives	Telling a story
THOUGHTS FEELINGS	
Why? How? So what?	What? When? Who? Where?

Figure 4.6 Reflection vs. description

The simplest way to think about description is that you are providing the what?, when?, who? and where?. This is the background for your reflection. Description is telling a story, and while you need to include some 'story telling' in order for your reflective writing to make sense, this should be just a small amount and only be at the start. In your reflective writing, you need to show that you have carefully considered thoughts, feelings and different perspectives to clearly demonstrate your reflective thinking. So, if you use description as an important, but small part of your reflective writing, it will help you to clearly show what you have learned. Figure 4.7 shows you where, using Borton's (1970) model of reflection, you can include description and where you should include reflection in order to demonstrate learning. When you are writing, remember that good reflective writing demonstrates reflective thinking, and showing your awareness of your learning is an important aspect of this.

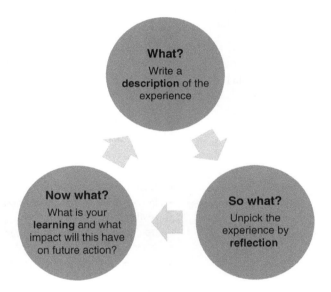

Figure 4.7   Description + reflection = learning

Source: Adapted from Borton (1970).

CONFIDENTIALITY

We have already mentioned confidentiality when we were talking about reflective diaries, but maintaining confidentiality is so important that it needs to be mentioned again. You must ensure that you maintain confidentiality at all times (NMC, 2018). Always remember to protect the patient's identity by changing their name, giving them a **pseudonym**, and stating this in your writing. In the same way that you need to change the patient's name, you need to do so for any other individuals you mention in your reflection, including the patient's family, nurses, other students or any other healthcare staff, and ensure you give them a pseudonym too. If the patient has a wife and three children, again you only need to mention these details if they play an important part in your reflection. Remember that you only need to include in your writing details about patients, other individuals and places, which are truly necessary, and never disclose their actual names or geographical location.

ADD A STRUCTURE AND PROMPTS

If we look back at all the aspects of reflective writing we have discussed so far, it is possible to identify a series of prompts to help when writing reflectively. If we add to this Borton's (1970) reflective model and identify the introductory, main body and concluding sections, we can create an effective structure to use for our reflective writing, as shown in Table 4.2.

Table 4.2   A structure for reflective writing

Section	Borton (1970) reflective model stage	What to include
Introduction *In all your writing, maintain confidentiality and use the first person.*	What? (Description and feelings)	• Introduce the writing by identifying what you are going to discuss and why. • Provide background information, but only give the necessary details. • Introduce the main points. • Refer back to the essay question (if relevant).
Main body	So what? (Evaluation and analysis)	• Identify 1-2 main topics. • Introduce the evidence and discuss how it relates to your experience. • Don't just describe what happened - reflect on why and how it happened. • Organise discussion into paragraphs that flow logically. • Be concise.
Conclusion	Now what? (Conclusion and action plan)	• Refer back to the essay question (if relevant). • Summarise the main points of your writing. • Identify and discuss your action plan.

In Table 4.2 we have used Borton's (1970) model of reflection, but it would be perfectly possible for you to transfer all the elements identified in the table to another reflective framework. See Chapter 10 for some ideas.

ACTIVITY 4.4

Refer back to Angus's reflection in Part A, using Table 4.2 as a checklist, and see whether he has used the structure and prompts we have created in his reflection.
   Can you identify any areas that Angus's work could be improved?

Check the activity answers at the end of the chapter to see if we agree.

Table 4.3 The master plan

Section	Borton's (1970) model of reflection – What? So what? What now?	Essential content	Reflection tips	Critical thinking tips
Remember you are writing your reflection in a 'formally informal' style, so use 'I, me, my' as appropriate in all sections. **Ensure that you maintain confidentiality at all times.** Introduction Introduce the writing by identifying what you are going to discuss and why. Provide only the necessary background information. Introduce the main points. Refer back to the essay question (if relevant).	What? Essential elements included in this stage: • critical incident • description This is the description of your critical incident. Here you write an overview of your experience describing: • What was the context for the experience? • Why is this experience important to you? • What happened? • How you were involved? • What exactly did you do? • What were your thoughts and feelings? • How did you respond to what happened?	A description of the experience. What were your feelings?	Focus on just one aspect of your experience so you can consider this issue in detail, rather than trying to consider lots of issues and not achieving any depth in your reflection. Make sure that your description is clear, so that the reader fully understands your experience. You are unlikely to be able to write a clear description on the first attempt at writing your experience down, so keep reading what you have written and refine it, until it says exactly what you want it to. At this point it can be useful to ask a friend to read what you have written and give you some feedback.	To get your reflection off to a good start: 1. ensure that you are not overly ambitious in what you chose to cover. Less really is more, as then you will be able to discuss issues in detail; 2. clearly identify what you are aiming to achieve. Jasper et al. (2013) suggest reflecting using SODA, which stands for **S**ignificance, **O**utcome, **D**escribable, **A**ction. While this can be used as a model in itself, if it is used in conjunction with other prompt questions, it can be useful in assisting critical thinking. The S, O and D part of SODA can be helpful for your critical thinking in this stage of Borton's (1970) model: Significance: Why was it significant? Why does it stand out in your mind? What is important about this incident? Outcome: What do you want to achieve as a result of this experience? What might you learn from it to help your practice? What might you learn about yourself? Describable: How can you describe it? What are the constraints? What may be the consequences? What are the ethical issues? What are the professional implications?

(Continued)

Table 4.3 (Continued)

Section	Borton's (1970) model of reflection – What? So what? What now?	Essential content	Reflection tips	Critical thinking tips
Main body **Identify one or two main topics.** **Introduce the evidence and discuss how it relates to your experience.** **Don't just describe what happened; reflect on why and how it happened.** **Organise discussion into paragraphs that flow logically.** **Be concise.**	So what? Essential elements included in this stage: • analysis; • interpretation; • perspective. This is where you break the experience down so you can question: • What was important in this experience? • What were your thoughts and feelings during the experience? • What theory relates to your experience? • What went well? • What could have gone better? • What were the consequences of your actions and beliefs? • Does the experience make you rethink your actions and beliefs? • What did the experience teach you? • How do your personal and professional values relate to the experience?	An evaluation of the experience. An analysis of the experience.	In this stage, the aim is to clearly demonstrate that you have carefully considered your experience and thought about the relationship between theoretical principles and practice. Your consideration needs to include discussion relating to the consequences of your actions and beliefs and, if relevant, those of any others involved. You need to provide evidence that you are aware of both your personal and professional values. To produce an effective reflection that achieves Goodman's Level 2 or 3, this section needs to use references to support the statements you are making. This will enable you to identify the reasoning behind and the evidence base of the actions you took.	This stage of the model has lots of opportunities to demonstrate critical thinking. Make sure that you use relevant evidence to support your writing so it is very clear how you know what you are stating. Get into the habit of supporting all the statements you make with evidence. 1. Identify and challenge any assumptions you made – this could relate to, for example, knowledge, values, actions, beliefs, emotions, the role of the patient, the role of the nurse, power, political issues, economic circumstances, decisions, etc. 2. What is actually happening in your experience? 3. Is there anything important missing? 4. What are the influences? 5. What if? 6. What was the aim of your actions? 7. What were your reasons for undertaking your actions? 8. Does the evidence support your reasons? 9. What are the assumptions behind your reasons? 10. What does all of this mean? 11. Have you considered all of the who, what, where, when, why, how questions? As mentioned in the previous section, Jasper et al. (2013) suggest that we can reflect using SODA. In this section, we could again consider the O and D of the model by discussing the following issues, but rather than repeating any previous discussion, develop this further.

Section	Borton's (1970) model of reflection – What? So what? What now?	Essential content	Reflection tips	Critical thinking tips
	• What would you do differently if you were faced with a similar situation – what would be the different actions or approaches you could take? • What is the significance of what happened? • What else do you need to consider to understand more fully what happened? • What sense can you make of this experience? • How did this experience influence or change you?		To achieve Goodman's Level 3, you also need to consider the broader social structures and forces, plus the wider influences of ethical and political decisions with regard to care delivery and practice.	Outcome: What did you achieve as a result of the experience? What did you learn from the experience to help your practice? What did you learn about yourself? Describable: How did you deal with the consequences of your actions? How did you deal with the ethical issues? How will the professional issues influence your future practice?
Conclusion **Refer back to the essay question (if relevant).** **Summarise the main points of your writing.** **Identify and discuss your action plan.**	**What now?** Essential element included in this stage: action. This where you put things back together – the synthesis – and relate this experience to your future, considering: • What do you need to do now? • What do I need to learn following my experience? • How are you going to do this?	A conclusion of all the points made. An action plan for future practice.	It is important in this section to demonstrate that you understand the need to know more and the actions you are going to take to achieve this.	In this section, you need to show that you have thought critically about what you can improve and/or how you will act differently as a result of your experience, again using the evidence to show how you have considered that this will demonstrate your critical thinking. Remember that you need to be: 1. objective, so while there may be some parts your actions you want to improve upon, there will also be some parts of your actions that went well; 2. honest about your thoughts, as this will enable you to both learn from your experience and learn about yourself. Again, we can use SODA (Jasper et al., 2013). In this section, we could again consider the A of the model by discussing the following issues: Action: What actions do you need to take? Who else can help you?

A MASTER PLAN

So far, throughout the first part of this book we have been working on developing your ability to produce an effective reflection. In Chapter 1 we discovered what reflection actually is, identified the tools we needed in order to reflect and introduced a reflective framework. In Chapter 2 we focused on producing a reflection and in Chapter 3 identified how we could include critical thinking in our reflection. In this chapter, we have been concentrating on how we actually write a reflection to ensure that it sounds knowledgeable but is still a personal interpretation of an experience. Table 4.3 (pp73–75) brings all these elements together, as it contains all the hints and tips we have highlighted in all the chapters so far. So, from now on, when you are reflecting, use Table 4.3 as your master plan to assist you to develop an effective reflection.

WORDS AND PHRASES

Although we now have a master plan for the structure and content of our reflection, there is one final but very important element that we need to consider. Throughout this chapter we have been working on our recipe for reflection. We have mixed all the ingredients, produced the cake and added the icing to it. What we are going to concentrate on now is the final decoration, which finishes the cake off with a flourish. In terms of reflective writing, the final decoration are the words and phrases you use. This is the *craft* of reflective writing. You have done all the planning and necessary thinking for your reflection; now you want to show this off to the best effect. Ensuring your writing style is correct is the final step.

ACTIVITY 4.5

Put this book down and, using your literature searching skills, find an academic article on a topic you are interested in. Read the first five paragraphs and then consider the following question:

What writing skills is the author applying to share their knowledge?

Check the activity answers at the end of the chapter to see if we agree.

In order to convey what you know and have the correct academic tone, it is important to be clear in your writing, and use words and phrases that the reader can readily understand. Some academic writing can be very difficult to comprehend, sounding as if the person writing it has swallowed a dictionary. You may have been reading a piece like this in Activity 4.5. This is not good academic writing, which should be both clear to understand and interesting to read. While you need to demonstrate that you have a good vocabulary when you are writing, there is no need to use words that are not common in general conversation. This also applies to the 'professional language' of specific terms we apply to, for example, patient care. Again, in your writing you should use those terms that are frequently used, but there is no need to use a complex term rather than a simple one.

There are a number of words and phrases that are useful when you are writing reflectively. If we think about the sections of your reflection in the same way they were identified in Table 4.2 – the introduction, the main body and the conclusion – it is possible to identify words and phrases that will be helpful in the main body and the conclusion. Due to the huge difference in what will be described in the introduction of a reflection, it is not possible to suggest words and phrases for that section. Within the introduction, however, do remember that if you are focusing on an event that happened in the past, you should use the past tense when describing it, and make sure that you have explained to the reader what you are going to focus on, so they understand this before they start to read your reflection in detail.

Table 4.4 provides many words and phrases you will find useful when writing the main body of your reflection and Table 4.5 identifies those that will be useful in the conclusion.

Table 4.4   Useful words and phrases for the main body

Section	Words and phrases			
Main body	**Evaluative phrases**			
(Evaluation and analysis of your experience)			aspect(s)	
			element(s)	
		meaningful	experience(s)	
		significant	issue(s)	
	For me the (most)	important	idea(s)	was (were)
		relevant		
		useful		
	arose from			
Learning	happened when			
	resulted from			
		Previously	thought (did not think)	
		At the time	felt (did not feel)	
		At first	knew (did not know)	
		Initially	noticed (did not notice)	
		Subsequently	questioned (did not question)	
		Later	realised (did not realise)	
Analytical phrases				
		might be	because of	
Alternatively	this	is perhaps	due to	
Equally		could be	explained by	
		is possibly	related to	
			similar to	
		This is	unlike	X because
(Un)like X this	reveals			
	demonstrates			

Source: Adapted from Hampton (2015), Academic Skills Unit, University of Portsmouth. Available at: https://capstone.unst.pdx.edu/sites/default/files/Reflective-writing---a-basic-intro_0.pdf#. Reproduced with kind permission of Julian Ingle, Head of the Academic Skills Unit at the University of Portsmouth.

Table 4.5 Useful words and phrases for the conclusion

Section	Words and phrases			
Conclusion	**Concluding phrases**			
(The conclusion of your experience and your plan for future actions)	Having	read experienced applied discussed analysed learned	I now	feel think realise wonder question know
			Additionally Furthermore Most importantly	I have learned that
	I have (not)	significantly slightly	developed improved	my skills in my understanding of my knowledge of my ability to
	This means that			
	This makes me feel			
	This knowledge	is	essential	to me personally because
	This understanding	could be	important	to me as a student because
	This skill	will be	useful	to me as a nurse because
	Action plan phrases			
	Because I	did not have not yet am not yet certain about am not yet confident about do not yet know do not yet understand	I now need to	
			As a next step I will	

Source: Adapted from Hampton (2015), Academic Skills Unit, University of Portsmouth. Available at: https://capstone.unst.pdx.edu/sites/default/files/Reflective-writing---a-basic-intro_0.pdf#. Reproduced with kind permission of Julian Ingle, Head of the Academic Skills Unit at the University of Portsmouth.

PROOFREADING

Once you have finished writing your reflection, you need to carefully **proofread** your work. This is a very important step in ensuring that your work has the correct writing style, sounds knowledgeable, has the correct academic tone, and that your spelling and grammar are correct. Make sure you don't spoil all the hard work you have put in so far by making errors in your spelling and grammar. Attention to detail is very important. If this is an aspect of writing you find difficult, ask a friend or relative to check your work for you. In fact, if you can find another person who is willing to read through your work, they can be really helpful by telling you whether they think what you have written flows well and makes sense. If you can't find another person to read through your work, put it away for a couple of days and then read it again. You will be amazed at how what you thought of as being perfect when you put it away isn't quite as clear as you want it to be and may still contain errors.

Reflective writing is a skill and, just like any skill, it will get better if you practise it. So, now you have a master plan and lots of useful phrases, it is over to you – get reflecting!

CONCLUSION

The ability to produce effective reflective writing is an important aspect of reflection for both formal and informal purposes. Reflective writing is how you demonstrate your ability to think reflectively, which is the true purpose of reflection. The process of reflective writing involves considering the meaning and impact of an experience, which enables learning about yourself both personally and professionally.

Although being able to write reflectively can at first seem challenging, there are a number of structures you can apply, plus hints and tips to use, which, when combined with practice, will support you to produce interesting and effective reflective writing.

GOING FURTHER

Bulman, C. and Schutz, S. (eds) (2013) *Reflective Practice in Nursing* (5th edn). London: Wiley-Blackwell. An excellent source of information for all matters relating to reflection. Chapter 3 focuses on reflective writing.

Donohoe, A. (2015) Reflective writing: Articulating an alternative pedagogy. *Procedia – Social and Behavioral Sciences*, 186: 800–4. A very interesting article that considers the evidence supporting the current approach to reflective writing in nurse education and suggests an alternative.

Writing reflectively. Go to: http://joyceshankarkay.blogspot.com/2016/05/reflective-writing-how-to.html. This is a short video explaining how to write reflectively, including what to write about, what to avoid writing about and the benefits of reflective writing.

—————————— ANSWERS TO ACTIVITIES ——————————

Activity 4.3

In Figure 4.5 Angus uses 'I, me and my' a total of 18 times. The extract from his reflection is only composed of 107 words, so 'I, me and my' make up a considerable percentage of the words he uses. His writing, however, does not sound like a letter because he isn't just describing his experience, but is evaluating and analysing it by relating it to being a volunteer teacher. Remember that when you are reflecting you need to do this, consider the 'why?', the 'how?' and the 'so what?'.

Activity 4.4

Comments on whether Angus achieved these elements in his reflection are italicised.

Table 4.6   **A structure for reflective writing (based on Angus's reflection)**

Section	Borton (1970) reflective model stage	What to include
In all of your writing maintain confidentiality *Yes, maintained confidentiality throughout.* and use the first person. *Yes.* **Introduction** *Used the first stage of Borton's model as an introduction to the work – he could have improved this by introducing what he was aiming to do before starting on the reflection.*	What? *Yes, used as a heading.* (Description and feelings) *Yes, described the situation very briefly and stated his feelings.*	• Introduce the writing by identifying what you are going to discuss and why. *Angus needed to do this.* • Provide necessary background information, but only give the necessary details. *Yes.* • Introduce the main points. *Yes.* • Refer back to the essay question (if relevant). *Not relevant.*
Main body *This is clear.*	So what? *Uses this as a heading, which is good because it clearly identifies how the reflective model is being used.* (Evaluation and analysis) *Angus tries to evaluate and analyse, but he doesn't write enough to achieve this in any detail.* *His evaluation and analysis could have been further improved by using some of the words and phrases associated with the section to help in the discussion.*	• Identify one or two main topics. *Focused upon just one topic, not knowing enough.* • Introduce the evidence and discuss how it relates to your experience. *Considered The Code (NMC, 2018) as evidence, but could have used more than just this to support the points he was making.* • Don't just describe what happened – reflect upon why and how it happened. *Considered the why and how but could have written more detail about this.* • Organise discussion into paragraphs which flow logically. *Two paragraphs which flow well.* • Be concise. *Yes.*

Section	Borton (1970) reflective model stage	What to include
Conclusion *This is clear.*	Now what? *Uses this as a heading which is good.* (Conclusion) *Clearly concludes the main points of his writing.* (Action plan) *Clearly identifies an action plan.*	• Refer back to the essay question (if relevant). *Not relevant.* • Summarise the main points of your writing. *Yes.* • Identify and discuss your action plan. *Yes.*

Activity 4.5

It is likely that the author of the article you are reading is applying all, or many of the following skills:

- The correct academic tone.
- Being clear in their writing.
- Using words and phrases that are readily understandable. While they will be demonstrating that they have a good vocabulary, they will not use words that are not in common usage in everyday or professional language.
- Their writing is interesting to read.
- Presenting ideas logically.
- Using evidence to support their discussion.
- Using correct punctuation, spelling and grammar.
- Avoiding unnecessary repetition.
- Being concise.

GLOSSARY

anecdotal   Subjective and like a story.

cognitively   Involving conscious intellectual activity.

introspection   The examination or observation of your mental and emotional processes.

personal pronouns   A pronoun is a word that can take the place of a noun; a personal pronoun is a pronoun that refers to a particular person, group or thing.

proofread   To read very carefully in order to identify any errors.

pseudonym   A fictitious name.

tone   The tone of your writing refers to how your voice sounds to the reader.

REFERENCES

Borton, T. (1970) *Reach, Touch and Teach*. London: Hutchinson.

Gibbs, G. (1988) *Learning by Doing: A Guide to Teaching and Learning Methods*. Oxford: Further Education Unit, Oxford Polytechnic.

Hampton, M. (2015) Reflective writing – a basic introduction. Available at: https://capstone.unst.pdx.edu/sites/default/files/Reflective-writing---a-basic-intro_0.pdf (accessed 23 August 2020).

Jasper, M., Rosser, M. and Mooney, G. (2013) *Professional Development, Reflection and Decision Making in Nursing and Health Care* (2nd edn). Chichester: John Wiley & Sons.

Nursing and Midwifery Council (NMC) (2018) *The Code.* London: NMC.

Public Health England (PHE) (2016) *The Eatwell Guide.* London: PHE.

Shankar-Kay, J. (2016) Reflecting is a 3 stage process. Available at: http://joyceshankarkay.blogspot.com/2016/05/reflective-writing-how-to.html (accessed 23 August 2020).

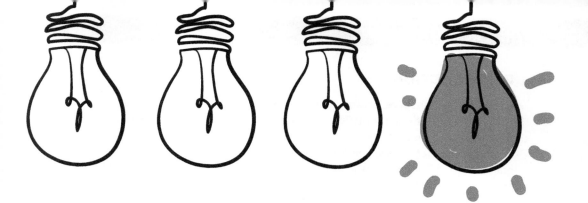

HOW CAN I REFLECT?

CATHERINE DELVES-YATES

5

> " Reflection – does it always have to be an essay? I know I have to do a formal written reflection for my assignment, but I find writing in this way dull and boring! I want to be able to reflect in a way that is more exciting!
>
> **Andy Tirepied, nursing student, mental health field** "

> " The biggest problem I have when reflecting is trying to see a situation from a different perspective. This is important if I want my reflection to be critical, but I find it so very difficult. How can I reflect in a way that helps me with this?
>
> **Lizzie Chandler, nursing student, child field** "

INTRODUCTION

When we think about reflection, often what we think about first is reflecting in a formal, written fashion – the sort of reflection that you will write for an assignment or revalidation. However, this isn't the only way to reflect and there are many other ways.

In this chapter we are going to consider the benefits and challenges of using formal written reflections and identify a criteria to consider when producing these as assignments or for revalidation. We are going to expand our knowledge of reflection by considering the differences between reflection on action and reflection in action, and then finally identify alternative, more creative, approaches to reflection, which Andy and Lizzie, who we met at the start of the chapter, might enjoy and find helpful.

—————————————— CHAPTER AIMS ——————————————

This chapter will enable you to:

- understand the benefits and challenges of using formal written reflection;
- consider the elements a formal written reflection needs to include;
- realise how your ability to reflect will develop with practice;
- appreciate the difference between reflection on action and reflection in action;
- comprehend the difference between reflection and mindfulness;
- identify differing and more creative ways to reflect.

FORMAL WRITTEN REFLECTIONS

As Andy highlights at the start of the chapter, when we talk about reflection, most of us will think of this as being a formal written piece, which usually applies a model to enable us to analyse and interpret our experience. In fact, if you look at previous chapters, you will see that this is exactly the approach we have been discussing. There is, however, good reason for this. Think about what prompted you to start reading this textbook. For most of us, the reason to start reading about how to reflect is because the deadline for an assignment where we need to produce a reflection or the date for our revalidation is rapidly approaching.

Associating reflection with assessments may cause us to see reflection as being a formal and rather sombre affair. There is an element of truth in this, as reflection is often a process we are required to undertake for official reasons, to prove our learning or ability to learn from experience. As nurses, however, we are responsible for delivering care to patients, so we need to be able to demonstrate that we are safe and competent in our practice. Producing a written reflection is a good way to do this and brings many benefits. There are also, however, some challenges, as Figure 5.1 outlines on the next page.

A TASK OR AN OPPORTUNITY TO LEARN?

As we have discussed in previous chapters, reflection provides you with an opportunity to consider how your personal experiences and observations influence both your thinking and acceptance of new ideas. Producing a written reflection is a particularly effective

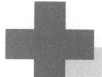

Benefits	Challenges
Writing a formal reflection:	Writing a formal reflection:
- has a positive impact upon learning from experiences;	- can be time-consuming;
- increases awareness of thoughts and actions;	- may not be enjoyable;
- results in a greater sense of self-awareness and mindfulness;	- may not be appropriate for a short, everyday reflections;
- identifies gaps in knowledge;	- can result in learning from reflection being overshadowed by the need to write formally;
- improves analytical skills;	- does not engage the creative parts of our brains;
- provides a strucutre to follow;	- may be thought to be too difficult;
- clearly focuses upon self improvement;	- can be seen as tedious and dull.
- enables you to pass assignments or achieve revalidation.	

Figure 5.1 Benefits and challenges of formal written reflections

---

ACTIVITY 5.1

Think about the benefits and challenges of formal written reflections identified in Figure 5.1.

- Can you think of any further benefits or challenges that could be added to the lists?
- How do you view formal written reflections? Do you think they help you to learn?

Check the activity answers at the end of the chapter to see if our thoughts are similar.

---

way to do this, as it provides a structure to follow which encourages you to explore your ideas and express your opinions based on relevant evidence. In this way, reflective writing can help you to improve your analytical skills because not only does it require you to identify your view, but more significantly, you have to consider how and why you think what you do. This 'reflective analysis' requires you to acknowledge that your thoughts are shaped by your assumptions and preconceived ideas. By working through this process, you can appreciate the ideas of others, notice how their assumptions and preconceived ideas may have shaped their thoughts, and recognise how your views support or oppose what you write.

Written reflections are used in many professions, such as healthcare and education, as a way to make connections between theory and practice. For example, when you are asked to reflect on an experience you have had with a patient, not only do you describe your experience, but more importantly you evaluate it based on evidence. In doing this, you consider a theory or approach in relation to your nursing care, which results in the evaluation of your knowledge and skills. The production of a formal written reflection encourages you to think about your choices, your actions, your successes and things that need to be improved. Theory, which when considered in isolation, can seem like an abstract **concept** when related to patients and your experience, becomes real. Reflecting on how you have applied theory assists you to make plans for improvement.

So, in consideration as to whether writing a formal reflection is a task or an opportunity for learning, it is both. It is true that producing a formal written reflection is time-consuming; it may not be enjoyable, the need to ensure that your written expression is clear and flows can be challenging, and the whole process can be tedious. However – and this is an important aspect – producing a formal written reflection does enable us to learn about ourselves as both nurses and individuals.

AN ASSESSMENT: MEETING THE CRITERIA

We often need to produce a written reflection as an assessment, either as a nursing student or registered nurse. While we will learn from writing the reflection, we also want to pass the assessment, so need to meet the identified criteria. The criteria may be something devised by the university you are studying at, or in the case of producing a reflection for revalidation, the criteria has been devised by the Nursing and Midwifery Council (NMC). The best starting point for any formal piece of written reflection is to make sure you understand the criteria. By doing this, you can ensure that what you produce is what is required, as otherwise, even if your writing is logical, well presented and carefully considered, you are unlikely to be successful.

ACTIVITY 5.2

Think about all you have read relating to reflection, writing formal reflections and any reflections you have written.

- Make a list of the elements of a formal written reflection that you think are important to include.
- Now turn your list into a 'marking criteria' by giving each item on your list a specific number of marks to be awarded. If you ensure that the total marks available in your marking criteria are 100, you will have identified a percentage mark for each item.

Check the activity answers at the end of the chapter to view my list and marking criteria to see if our thoughts are similar.

If we consider what all universities and the NMC feel should be included in a formal written reflection, while there might be some slight differences, there would also be a great deal of agreement.

A formal written reflection would need to apply a reflective model such as Borton (1970), the one Angus uses in Part A. The writing would need to include a clear and detailed description of the experience, which is the focus of the reflection. The writer would have to demonstrate that they were self-aware. It would be expected that within the reflection appropriate theories, concepts and strategies were made relevant to the nursing care being considered and that the work was well presented. There would need to be critical and analytical discussion throughout the reflection, although this would be less for a nursing student at the start of their programme than it was for a final-year nursing student or a registered nurse. All the statements made and the views discussed would need to be supported with evidence, and references to this evidence would need to follow the format identified by the university. Finally, the reflection would need to be written clearly and use an appropriate academic writing style.

ACTIVITY 5.3

Angus's reflection

Read the reflection written by Angus in Part A.

- Use either the marking criteria you devised in Activity 5.2, or use the one I shared in the answer to the activity 5.2, to 'mark' Angus's reflection.
- What aspects did Angus do well in and what feedback would you give him for his future development?

Check the activity answers at the end of the chapter to see if our thoughts are similar.

If we look in detail at Angus's reflection, he applied Borton's model (1970), but he could have improved this by highlighting in more detail his rationale for choosing this model. He needed to say more than just that it was the easiest to understand. Angus could also have outlined the aim of each of the stages of the model. Saying that the aim of the first stage was to describe the experience, the second stage aimed to enable making sense of the experience and the final stage focused on plans for what to do next, would have provided clear evidence that Angus understood the model he was applying. He could also have been more **explicit** in the final stage as to what exactly his planned future actions were.

Angus made a good attempt to describe the experience he was reflecting on, but he could have made this more detailed and focused. He needed to describe a specific incident, which made him realise how unconfident he was feeling, rather than a more general approach.

In his reflection, Angus showed some self-awareness. His reflection would have been improved, however, if he had written explicitly about this. Angus could have mentioned that one of the benefits of reflection is learning about yourself; he could have defined the term 'self-awareness' and explained exactly what he had learnt about himself.

An important area for improvement in Angus's reflection is in applying theory or concepts to nursing practice. Angus makes a serious omission when he doesn't do this. One of the important benefits of reflection is linking theory with practice, so this is something that must be included. Angus does highlight future actions, but again these needed to be more detailed.

Angus presents his reflection well, and the material discussed is considered in a logical fashion.

Being critical and analytical is an important area where Angus's reflection needs development. We must remember, however, that this is the first reflection that Angus has written; being both critical and analytical are skills that need practice.

Angus also needs to develop his ability to support the points he makes with appropriate evidence, which means making reference to relevant literature, such as research-based journal articles, professional standards and clinical practice guides. In this reflection, Angus has only made one reference to *The Code* (NMC, 2018); he needs to use more references than this. When using references, Angus has applied an accepted reference format when he refers to *The Code*, but he needs to include a reference list at the end of his reflection.

In general, Angus's reflection is well written, his spelling is correct and he hasn't made any grammatical errors. However, his writing style is 'chatty'. It is important to remember that although reflections are written in the first person (using I, me, my and referring to yourself), they still need to be written in an academic style. This involves including evidence and being critical and analytical, as well as being clear, concise, focused and structured. Academic writing, even when written in the first person, has a formal tone and style; it is not written in the same way as a letter or an email, for example.

In summary, Angus has made a good first attempt at a formal written reflection; he is clearly starting to develop his skills. As he progresses through his nursing programme, practises reflective writing and becomes more proficient, his writing skills will improve.

To see how reflective writing improves if you practise, read Gail's reflection in the case study below.

CASE STUDY 5.1: GAIL'S REFLECTION

Gail Selby is an adult nursing student in the last year of her programme. For her final assignment she was asked to produce 'A structured reflection demonstrating critical self-awareness relating to professional development and academic progression during the final year of the nursing programme'. This is what she wrote.

INTRODUCTION

Self-awareness is a dynamic process involving the analysis and evaluation of thoughts, feelings and values to gain personal insight (Eckcroth-Bucher, 2010). It aids understanding of personal strengths and weaknesses (Rasheed, Younas and Sundus, 2019) and facilitates the development of critical thinking and decision-making skills (Han and Kim, 2016). Reflective practice is a recognised strategy for self-awareness development (Elcock and Shapcott, 2018) and an essential part of the learning process to help inform practice (Thorpe and Delves-Yates, 2018). This reflection critically appraises my professional and academic progression focusing on planning, prioritising and delegation. Borton's (1970) What?, So what?, Now what? has been used because its simplistic framework suits the reflective subject.

WHAT?

Time-management has been essential for my professional role and academic study. Prioritising, managing time, staff and resources effectively to maintain safety are key requisites within *The Code* (NMC, 2018). My placements have required me to take greater responsibility to manage mine and others' time, as well as planning and prioritising patient care. My placement in cardiology involved taking the lead in providing care for up to ten patients simultaneously, working closely with my placement supervisor and health care assistants (HCAs). Academically, completing two written assignments and preparing two seminars, one with a fellow student, while balancing work and family life required effective planning.

Although time-management was effective in my academic study, it presented challenges within my professional role.

SO WHAT?

I demonstrated effective time-management when working on academic assignments by creating a detailed study plan to meet deadlines while allowing adequate personal time. I felt my time-management skills would transfer easily to my professional role. However, I struggled with the handover of care affecting my ability to plan and prioritise the management of my patients; consequently, my practice supervisor needed to step in and help. Handover of care transfers professional responsibility and accountability (Merten, 2017), and is identified as a major risk point impacting on patient safety and clinical outcomes (Bruton, et al., 2016). SBAR (situation, background, assessment, recommendation) provides a framework for handing over information clearly and concisely (NHS Improvement, 2018), yet miscommunication remains a leading cause for adverse events (Eggins and Slade, 2015). The amount of domain-specific language and abbreviations was difficult to follow. Subsequently, I missed much of the patient information and therefore lacked understanding of their care. I felt embarrassed that I was unable to follow handover and lost confidence in my abilities. Through my academic study, I developed research skills and used these to improve my confidence and knowledge on cardiac conditions and management, therapeutic procedures and recovery protocols and standard cardiac abbreviations. Making use of systematic searches, the library and the Intranet ensured the most up-to-date information to facilitate best practice. Consequently, I was able to plan and prioritise patient care successfully.

Critical thinking developed through written assignments has been a key factor in developing planning and prioritising skills in practice. For example, I prioritised a patient on an insulin infusion with uncontrolled blood sugar over one requiring intravenous antibiotics. Administering the antibiotics 30 minutes late would not worsen their condition, but the continuing high blood sugar could cause significant harm. Prioritising is a dynamic process open to ongoing re-evaluation (Castledine, 2013). I used ward routines such as drug rounds and patient accountabilities to assess current patient care, and plan and reprioritise accordingly.

Delegating is essential to meet all the patients' needs, as caring for many patients simultaneously can lead to conflicting demands on time (Lake, Moss and Duke, 2009). Leading the team, I lacked authority and confidence in delegating, particularly when working with staff who presented a 'challenge'. Consequently, I tried to do everything myself. Additionally, I was unsure regarding HCA roles and competency levels. However, after discussing it with my practice supervisor, I recognised that some aspects of patient care were being

(Continued)

delayed or neglected because I was not delegating. Delegation is a complex nursing skill (Hasson, McKenna and Keeney, 2013), but working collaboratively aids the process, ensuring that workload is distributed effectively to manage changing priorities and provide safe care (Potter et al., 2010; Magnusson et al., 2017). Working in isolation can result in poor communication and inadequate supervision of HCAs (Johnson et al., 2015).

To manage my concerns around authority, my practice supervisor ensured staff working with me were aware that I was managing patient care. This strategy was effective as it immediately boosted my confidence knowing staff would expect me to delegate. Collaborative working relies on mutual information sharing to ensure continuity of patient care (CQC, 2013); therefore, I spent time helping the HCAs at the start of the shift. This allowed me to discuss the plan, confirm their competency level and delegate any additional responsibilities. I 'checked-in' with them at regular intervals to ensure they were managing their workload and to update them on any changes to the plan. Additionally, this allowed me to ensure they were appropriately supervised. I feel this approach helped develop a working relationship based on mutual trust and further increased my confidence around delegation. However, there were staff who presented a 'challenge' and I undertook tasks I should have delegated to avoid conflict.

NOW WHAT?

This reflection has considered my academic and professional progression, focusing on the challenges in planning, prioritising and delegating patient care. It considers how my lack of knowledge, authority and confidence in delegating, particularly with 'challenging' staff, affected effective performance in these areas. Recognising my future role as a registered nurse highlights the need for further development.

Self-efficacy relates to an individual's belief in their own ability to succeed in a situation (Bandura, 1977); developing greater self-belief will help in unknown or stressful situations. Therefore, I need to undertake practical experiences of situations I fear rather than avoiding them to help gain a sense of achievement leading to greater self-efficacy. Support and encouragement from nursing colleagues is linked to improving confidence (Mason and Davies, 2013); therefore, I can access this during times of self-doubt. It is important that I appear confident, as acting as a role-model, displaying positive professional behaviours, can be influential on others (Major, 2019). It can develop confidence and establish trust and respect from the team (Doody and Doody, 2012), which in turn can promote self-confidence.

I have developed effective academic skills that have underpinned my nursing practice and will continue to use these to inform and develop further. Increasing my nursing knowledge and expertise through experiential learning and reflective practice will be instrumental in my continuing professional development.

REFERENCES

Bandura, A. (1977) 'Self-efficacy: toward a unifying theory of behavioural change', Psychological Review, 84(2), pp. 191-215.

Borton, T. (1970) Reach, Touch and Teach. London, Hutchinson.

Bruton, J., Norton, C., Smyth, N., Ward, H. and Day, S. (2016) 'Nurse handover: patient and staff experiences'. *British Journal of Nursing*, 25(7), pp. 386-393.

Care Quality Commission (CQQ) (2013) *Raising Standards, Putting People First: Our Strategy for 2013 to 2016*. Available at: www.cqc.org.uk/sites/default/files/documents/20130503_cqc_strategy_2013_final_cm_tagged.pdf (accessed 17 August 2020).

Castledine, G. (2013) 'Prioritizing care is an essential nursing skill'. *British Journal of Nursing*, 11(14).

Doody, O. and Doody, C.M. (2012) 'Transformational leadership in nursing practice'. *British Journal of Nursing*, 21(20), pp. 1212-1218.

Eckroth-Bucher, M. (2010) 'Self-awareness: a review and analysis of a basic nursing concept'. *Advances in Nursing Science*, 33(4), pp. 297-309.

Eggins, S. and Slade, D. (2015) 'Communication in clinical handover: improving the safety and quality of the patient experience'. *Journal of Public Health Research*, 4(666), pp. 197-199.

Elcock, K. and Shapcott, J. (2018) 'Core communication skills', in Delves-Yates, C. (ed.) *Essentials of Nursing Practice* (2nd edn). London, Sage Publications Ltd, pp. 219-232.

Han, S. and Kim, S. (2016) 'An integrative literature review on self-awareness education/training programs in the nursing area'. *Perspectives in Nursing Science*, 13(2), pp. 59-69.

Hasson, F., McKenna, H.P. and Keeney, S. (2013) 'Delegating and supervising unregistered professionals: the student nurse experience'. *Nurse Education Today*, 33(3), pp. 229-235.

Johnson, M., Magnusson, C., Allan, H., Evans, K., Ball, E., Horton, K., Curtis, K. and Westwood, S. (2015) 'Doing the writing and working in parallel: how distal nursing affects delegation and supervision in the emerging role of the newly qualified nurse'. *Nurse Education Today*, 35(2), pp. e29-e33.

Lake, S., Moss, C. and Duke, J. (2009) 'Nursing prioritization of the patient need for care: a tacit knowledge embedded in the clinical decision-making literature'. *International Journal of Nursing Practice*, 15(5).

Magnusson, C., Allan, H., Horton, K., Johnson, M., Evans, K. and Ball, E. (2017) 'An analysis of delegation styles among newly qualified nurses'. *Nursing Standard*, 31(25), pp. 46-53.

Major, D. (2019) 'Developing effective nurse leadership skills'. *Nursing Standard*, 34(6), pp. 61-66.

Mason, J. and Davies, S. (2013) 'A qualitative evaluation of a preceptorship programme to support newly qualified midwives'. *Evidence Based Midwifery*, 11(3), pp. 94-98.

Merten, H. (2017) 'Safe handover'. *BMJ*, 359(4328), pp. 1-5.

NHS Improvement (2018) *SBAR communication tool – situation, background, assessment, recommendation*. Available at: https://improvement.nhs.uk/documents/2162/sbar-communication-tool.pdf (accessed 17 August 2020).

NMC (2018) *The Code*. NMC.

Potter, P., Deshields, T. and Kuhrik, M. (2010) 'Delegation practices between registered nurses and nursing assistive personnel'. *Journal of Nursing Management*, 18(2), pp. 157-165.

(Continued)

Rasheed, S.P., Younas, A. and Sundus, A. (2019) 'Self-awareness in nursing: a scoping review'. *Journal of Clinical Nursing*, 28, pp. 762-774.

Thorpe, G. and Delves-Yates, C. (2018) 'Core academic skills', in Delves-Yates, C. (ed.) *Essentials of Nursing Practice*, 2nd edn. London: Sage Publications Ltd, pp. 35-52.

ACTIVITY 5.4

Read the reflection written by Gail in the case study.

- Using the same marking criteria as you used to mark Angus's reflection, mark Gail's reflection.
- In what areas did Gail do well?
- What are the differences between Gail and Angus's reflections?

Check the activity answers at the end of the chapter to see if our thoughts are similar.

Reflection is the same as any other skill: the more you practise it, the better you get. As soon as you start reading Gail's reflection, it becomes clear that she has more nursing experience and has written more reflections than Angus. This is, of course, what we would expect, as Angus is at the start of his studies as a nursing student and Gail is at the end of hers.

Gail clearly applies Borton's reflective model, the same model as Angus did, and Gail's writing leads us through the stages effectively. In a similar way to Angus, Gail could have provided a more extensive rationale to support the choice of model, and an indication of the aim of the three stages would have provided evidence that she had a detailed understanding of the model. The question asked in Gail's assessment is challenging, as it actually asks her to reflect on two differing situations. Gail has dealt with this effectively by considering the common 'themes' linking these situations in her reflection.

Two areas where Gail's reflection is strong is in the consideration of self-awareness. This is explicitly addressed and demonstrated, as is the application of theory, concepts and strategies.

The presentation of Gail's reflection is very good visually, plus the material progresses in a logical fashion, and the reflection is well written with a good academic style throughout. There is also a consistently good level of critical consideration of the issues highlighted, with a sound level of analysis. Finally, Gail has used the evidence very well to support the views she discusses, and the reference format she applies is correct throughout.

In summary, Gail has produced an excellent reflection; she has clearly worked hard during the nursing programme to develop her skills. These skills will prove a very useful support to her ongoing development as she progresses in her new role as a registered nurse.

In her reflection, Gail has shown us how we can effectively reflect after our actions. However, this is not the only way to reflect – it is also possible to reflect while we are in the course of our actions.

REFLECTION ON ACTION AND REFLECTION IN ACTION

When we have been considering reflection so far in this textbook, what we have been doing is looking back on an experience and **retrospectively** contemplating what we have done. However, this should not be thought of as the only type of reflection. Schön (1991) presented the concept that there are differing types of reflection. Two of these are reflection on action, which is what we have been concentrating on, and reflection in action, which occurs during an experience. The features of both of these types of reflection are highlighted in Figure 5.2.

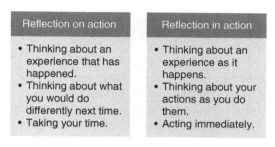

Reflection on action	Reflection in action
• Thinking about an experience that has happened. • Thinking about what you would do differently next time. • Taking your time.	• Thinking about an experience as it happens. • Thinking about your actions as you do them. • Acting immediately.

Figure 5.2   Reflection on action and reflection in action

We can see from Figure 5.2 that there are considerable differences in approach. All the chapters so far have been focused on developing reflection on action skills. We have been looking back on an experience, subjecting it to a **cognitive** post-mortem by interpreting and analysing the information we recall. From this, we have translated the information gained from the experience into learning, both about ourselves and the practice of nursing.

Reflection in action, on the other hand, provides us with the ability to think about what we are doing while we are doing it. This is important because it enables us to alter what we are doing as we are doing it. Although reflection in action is frequently associated with experienced practitioners, it is a useful approach for anyone to use. This is especially important if we find ourselves in a situation where an experience is not progressing in the way we wish, or if we are doing something for the first time. Reflection in action enables us to improve the outcome of the experience we are participating in, rather than reflection on action which enables us to improve the outcome of an experience in the future. This makes reflection in action a very useful tool to use in nursing, where we often need to react to an event as it occurs, rather than having the luxury of being able to think about what happened and make plans for future changes.

ACTIVITY 5.5

Read Billy and Charlie's experiences below. Then decide:

- Which describes reflection on action?
- Which describes reflection in action?

(Continued)

Check the activity answers at the end of the chapter to see if we agree.

Billy

Billy is in a lecture but keeps being distracted by thinking about what to have for lunch. He wants to get the most from the lecture, so realises that he needs to find a way to help him focus. Billy decides the best course of action is to make notes of the key points of the lecture.

Charlie

Charlie realises that often after a lecture he can't remember what was covered. He decides in future to:

1.   find out some information about the lecture topic in advance;
2.   write down some questions he wants to find the answers for;
3.   make notes during the lecture to help him focus;
4.   arrange to go for a coffee after the lecture with a couple of friends who are also on the course to talk about what they have learnt;
5.   keep a file of lecture notes and any handouts.

The clear difference between reflection in action and reflection on action is timing. Reflection in action is a rapid **intuitive** process that is led by the person involved in the event. Reflection on action is a slower, deliberate process that is led by a model of reflection. The need to act rapidly and intuitively without a model to follow is why reflection in action is frequently associated with experienced practitioners. Logical rather than emotional thinking, plus the application of knowledge and previous experience are all key factors in reflection in action. However, the more proficient you become with reflection on action, the better you will become at reflection in action.

ACTIVITY 5.6

Reflection in action is a skill and will improve if you practise. When you next find yourself in a situation where you want to change the outcome, as Billy did when he was in a lecture, practise reflection in action. After the experience, make a note what happened and consider:

*   How did your reflection in action change the outcome of the experience?
*   What have you learnt from this experience which you can apply to your next reflection in action?

There is no definitive answer for this activity.

MINDFULNESS, REFLECTION AND NURSING CARE

Johns (2017) highlights that reflective practice ranges from reflection as an act to 'mindful practice' as a way of being. When he mentions 'mindful practice', this raises the question whether he is identifying a connection between reflection and mindfulness.

To investigate this further, the distinguishing features of reflection and mindfulness are outlined in Figure 5.3.

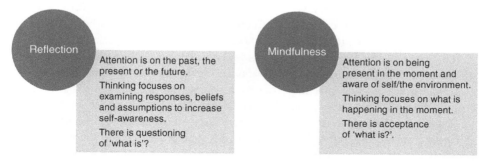

Figure 5.3   Distinguishing features of reflection and mindfulness

Considering Figure 5.3, it is possible to differentiate mindfulness from reflection through differences in timing and the focus of the thinking. The greatest difference is that reflection involves questioning, while mindfulness involves acceptance. So, when Johns (2017) refers to mindful practice, what he is saying is that reflection enables us to be mindful of ourselves, either within or after an experience. What he is indicating is that reflection develops our self-awareness and if we use every experience as a window through which we can view ourselves, reflection can become a way of being. He is not linking reflection with the practice of mindfulness.

This is not to say, however, that mindfulness has no place in nursing care. Learning how to be mindful as a nurse has been linked with the development of greater self-kindness and an increase in the ability to care for yourself.

DIFFERENT WAYS TO REFLECT

At the start of the chapter, Andy asked whether there were any ways other than formal written reflections he could use to reflect because he wanted to find a way that was more exciting. Formal reflective writing is not the only approach and there are other more creative ways to reflect on experiences.

Reflecting 'with yourself'

It can be helpful to reflect by 'thinking something through in your head' or by having a reflective conversation with yourself. Talking out loud is often a very good approach to clarifying the meaning of what you are thinking and focusing your thoughts on a few matters, rather than all the ideas running through your mind.

While this 'thinking something through in your head' or talking to yourself out loud does share many features with reflection, we need to be aware of the differences.

Reflection is a process undertaken with a specific purpose; 'thinking something through in your head' or talking to yourself out loud tends not to be, unless you apply a specific structure. If you want to try such an approach, following the stages of your favourite reflective model will help you to consider an experience in a critical fashion and turn your thinking into reflection.

It may also be valuable to capture your reflective conversation with yourself, using either an audio or video recording. Being able to watch or listen to your recording will allow you to consider in more detail what you said, develop your ideas and maybe even come to a new conclusion. You might then decide to use your video or audio recording as the focus of a more formal written reflection, or just keep your recordings as a personal record.

It is, of course, possible to share your recorded reflections with others. You may choose to do this in order to gain the perspective of another individual who you think could further assist your development. If we think back to the question Lizzie asked at the start of the chapter, she would find this approach helpful. Do remember, however, that you must at all times abide by *The Code* (NMC, 2018) and maintain confidentiality. Also, think carefully about the content of the recording and whether it is appropriate to share. You should never feel that you have to share anything you are uncomfortable with others knowing, and in the same way do not share something that is too personal for the individual seeing or hearing it.

Reflecting with others

There can be great value in having reflective conversations with others. It may actually be that you have already experienced this approach without realising it – see Table 5.1 for ways in which reflecting with others can take place, and the benefits and challenges of each approach.

Being creative

You can also be creative when you reflect. We have already considered recording audio or video reflections. It is possible to turn these into a blog or vlog; once again, you would need to ensure that you maintain confidentiality and uphold all aspects of *The Code* (NMC, 2018).

Other ways would be to keep a reflective diary which could be written or recorded, or more creatively write a poem, a song or a letter, do a painting, a drawing, use sketchnotes or keep a scrapbook. Again, in each of these reflective methods, we must ensure that we maintain confidentiality and uphold all aspects of *The Code* (NMC, 2018).

Two of my favourite ways to reflect creatively are to use sketchnotes or to write a letter.

Using sketchnotes

Sketchnoting is a form of notetaking, which combines words and pictures. It is the combination of writing and drawing that makes this an effective method for either taking notes or reflecting on an experience. The focus in sketchnoting is on ideas, not on the artistic merit of what you produce. I am not a gifted artist, but frequently find myself 'doodling' and drawing simple images while I am listening. If this describes you, and even if it doesn't, give sketchnoting a reflection a try. Figure 5.4 gives you an example of how you can do this, as it shows Angus's reflection, from Part A, using sketchnotes.

Table 5.1 Reflecting with others

Type of reflective conversation	What can be offered?	Benefits	Challenges
With a more experienced individual.	In a reflective conversation they will assist you to:	Gain the perspective of another individual.	In a formal relationship you may not feel able to share all the concerns or information relating to an experience.
With a supervisor, line manager, practice supervisor/assessor, university lecturer or clinical supervisor, for example.	• critically reflect upon your experience;	No need to concentrate on writing or following a model.	
You have a formal relationship with these individuals due to your role as either a registered nurse or student.	• identify an action plan and support you to achieve it.	Share concerns and identify a plan of action. This can be a good way to achieve your reflexive discussion for revalidation.	
With a mentor.	In a reflective conversation they will assist you to:		Confidentiality, and remember you must abide by all aspects of *The Code* (NMC, 2018).
Your relationship with a mentor will be informal.	• critically reflect on your work/educational experiences;		Although this is an informal relationship, you still may not feel able to share all the concerns or information relating to an experience.
A mentor can be anyone with more experience than you. Typically, they will be an expert in an area where you wish to develop your skills.	• identify an action plan.		
With a peer.	Conversations with friends are not always reflective, but they can be if your friend asks for the rationale behind an action. The simplest way to do this is just by asking 'why?'.	You may feel able to be completely honest with a friend.	Confidentiality, and remember you must abide by all aspects of *The Code* (NMC, 2018).
With a friend.		A friend will know you well and is likely to understand your feelings.	You need to agree and uphold boundaries – for example, is it acceptable for what you have discussed to be shared with others? A peer may not have the knowledge to understand the issues you are discussing.

(Continued)

Table 5.1 (Continued)

Type of reflective conversation	What can be offered?	Benefits	Challenges
		You will benefit from being able to see the experience you are discussing from the perspective of another. If your friend is suitably registered, this can be a good way to achieve your reflexive discussion for revalidation.	When conversing with a peer, rather than someone with greater experience than you, it can be tempting to think that their views, if they are not the same as yours, are wrong. Always try to find out why others have another perspective by respectful questioning and learn from differences.
With a critical friend. This is a peer who you ask for feedback and who questions you on your actions and your plans.	In a reflective conversation they will ask you to provide a rationale for your actions by asking 'why?'.	Being able to reflect with a critical friend you trust, who is able to ask effective questions, offers constructive feedback and has a sound understanding of the issues you are discussing, will enable you to develop both your personal and professional knowledge. You will benefit from being able to see the experience you are discussing from the perspective of another. If your critical friend is suitably registered, this can be a good way to achieve your reflexive discussion for revalidation.	
In a group. A group can be used to reflect on a shared experience, such as patient care or a placement.	In a reflective conversation, other group members will ask you to provide a rationale for your actions by asking 'why?'.	A group can be seen as a number of critical friends, so this is an excellent way to benefit from the perspectives of many others.	Confidentiality, and remember you must abide by all aspects of The Code (NMC, 2018). You need to agree and uphold boundaries – for example, is it acceptable for what you have discussed to be shared with others? Other group members may not have the knowledge to understand the issues you are discussing. When conversing in a group, if only one individual has a different perspective from the rest of the group, it can be tempting to think that their view is wrong. Always try to find out why others have another perspective by respectful questioning and learn from differences.

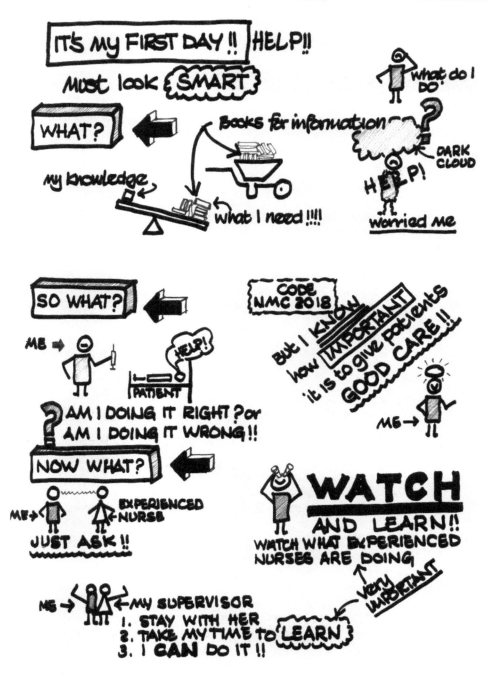

Figure 5.4 Angus's sketchnote reflection

Writing a letter

Writing your reflection in the format of a letter can be a really effective and creative way of reflecting. This is especially so if you are at the end of a programme of learning, as you can look back on what you have achieved and set out what actions you need to take for the future. This is exactly the approach that Coral took (see Case study 5.2 below).

CASE STUDY 5.2: CORAL'S LETTER

In January 2014, Coral Drane was a final-year adult field nursing student, writing the last reflection of her nursing programme. Coral decided to write the reflection in the form of a letter. This is what she wrote.

INTRODUCTION

This is my final reflection and I am both excited and sad at the prospect. For this reflection I have decided to use a letter format, as suggested by Bulman and Shulz (2013), and within this letter I will loosely use the framework of Boud et al. (1985) as I feel it will allow me the opportunity of "returning to my experiences" as advocated by the model (Boud et al., 1985, p. 27), "attending to [my] feelings" and "re-evaluating experience[s]" (Boud et al., 1985, p. 29–30). I will not use headings, as they will disturb the flow of the letter.

[Words in square brackets are my additions.]

8 January 2014

Dear Lecturer

I am writing to you to give you an update on my experiences during my nursing programme and to let you know how I have progressed during this final year, my main achievements and my development needs for the future. In this letter I will reflect on experiences, express how I feel about them and what I have learned from them.

My experiences in this final year have been extremely varied and valuable. The first part of my final year, term A, was about medical nursing, and I loved the enquiry-based learning (EBL) sessions that we prepared and delivered; our facilitator was very strict and required a high standard, which we all rose to. She also asked us to continually update the fictitious patient notes on a weekly basis and randomly checked them as if she were a Care Quality Commission inspector, which ensured that we kept up to date and gave us a taste of quality processes. My medical placement that followed was also extremely good and I gained much learning about cardiology nursing.

During term A, I also took part in an inter-professional learning conference on alcohol abuse, and prepared a poster with a medical student for the conference poster competition focusing on how the Gold Standards Framework (2012) could be used generically to support patients with alcohol issues. The poster won the local competition and then a national competition run by the Centre for the Advancement of Inter-professional Learning. It was excellent working with the medical student to produce the poster and we were extremely pleased to win both the local and national competitions. Additionally, during term A we wrote a critical incident analysis assignment. For this I used Carper's 'Patterns of Knowing' (Carper, 1978), which I found an extremely effective framework for deep, wide-ranging reflection, and the assignment also helped to increase my understanding of patient safety.

In the second term of the year, term B, we focused on emergency/critical care. Again, I found the EBL sessions challenging and rewarding, enjoying the resource preparation and presentations. The lectures were also extremely valuable and prepared us effectively for the practice element of the term that followed. My critical care placement was rich in terms of learning, particularly relating to the use of the ABCDE assessment process (Resuscitation Council, 2005), and the time I spent with the paramedics taught me, crucially, that I can remain calm and contribute in a crisis situation.

Finally, in the last term of the year, term C, we developed our nursing management, and I have found that my management skills are growing. I am gradually feeling more confident in terms of my prioritisation of care, management of groups of patients and my ability to delegate. I also completed my dissertation during term C and found the whole process challenging, interesting and rewarding; writing about handover has definitely heightened my awareness of the absolutely central importance of effective communication processes.

Considering my overall feelings related to this year, as suggested by the Boud et al. (1985) reflective model, emotionally, I have for the most part been extremely happy and feel so lucky to have had this opportunity to become a nurse at this mature stage in my life. Re-evaluating the experiences, at times I know that I lack confidence in my ability when on placement; this has been a thread running through the whole of my three years. I feel that it is good that I lack confidence in some instances, as it means that I will never work beyond my limitations, in line with the NMC *Code* (2008). However, I also know that if I lack confidence, it might affect my development, through decreasing my self-esteem and therefore impacting on my assertiveness and ability to cope (Rana and Upton, 2009). I am also aware that at times I do lack assertiveness. I will endeavour, therefore, when I become aware that I am losing confidence or lacking assertiveness, to seek appropriate support and guidance from a mentor and participate in appropriate continuous professional development (CPD).

If I were to consider now where my competence lies as a nurse related to Benner's (1982) stages of development, I feel that I am at advanced beginner stage. This is especially so in relation to management and some nursing skills that I have not had significant opportunity to practise. I will therefore work hard to grow to a competent level once registered, through on-going practice and relevant CPD. I feel, however, that in the areas of communication, connecting with patients (Halldorsdottir, 2008), empathising and my 'therapeutic use of self' (Carper, 1978), I am at a competent level and intend to develop to a higher level as my experience in nursing extends.

To conclude, as I stand on the brink of registration as a nurse, I feel a mixture of enthusiasm and trepidation. I have enjoyed being a nursing student and gained so much learning from the course, placements and the many reflections.

(Continued)

This experience has given me the fundamental tools to enable me to be a compassionate, effective staff nurse, and a mentor of the future.

Thank you for your continuous support throughout the programme.

Yours faithfully,
Coral

REFERENCES

Benner, P. (1982) 'From novice to expert', *American Journal of Nursing*, 82(3), pp. 402–407.

Boud, D., Keogh, R. and Walker, D. (1985) *Reflection: Turning Experience into Learning*. London: Kogan Page Ltd.

Bulman, C. and Schulz, S. (2013) *Reflective Practice in Nursing* (5th edn). Chichester: John Wiley & Sons Ltd.

Carper, B. (1978) 'Fundamental patterns of knowing in nursing'. *Advances in Nursing Science*, 1(1), 13–23.

Gold Standards Framework (2012) *The Gold Standards Framework*. Available at: www.goldstandardsframework.org.uk (accessed 8 January 2014).

Halldorsdottir, S. (2008) The dynamics of the nurse–patient relationship: introduction of a synthesised theory from the patient's perspective. *Scandinavian Journal of Caring Science*, 22: 643–52.

NMC (2008) *The Code*. London, NMC.

Rana, D. and Upton, D. (2009) *Psychology for Nurses*. Harlow: Pearson Education Ltd.

Resuscitation Council (2005) *A Systematic Approach for the Acutely Ill*. Available at: www.resus.org.uk/pages/alsabcde.htm (accessed 8 January 2014).

As you read Coral's letter, what stands out as particularly effective is her careful consideration of the range of experience she has been involved in during her final year and her ability to learn from each of these. She demonstrates that she has increased her self-awareness and identifies clear actions based on this knowledge. Throughout the letter, Coral has considered relevant evidence for her statements and been critically analytical in her approach. It is unusual for a letter to come with a list of references, but as Coral submitted this as a formal reflection for an assessment, it was necessary. You may think that this is a format you could use, maybe to fulfil an assignment or to personally reflect on an experience and identify areas that you would like to develop in the future.

CONCLUSION

When we think about reflection, we often think about a process involving writing a formal reflection. There is good reason for our thoughts: this approach to reflection is an excellent way to link theory to practice, prove our learning and demonstrate that we can learn from experience and are self-aware. Such an approach, however, may not be one we all enjoy, especially for informal, personal reflections.

Whatever approach we use when reflecting, if our resulting work is being used for an assessment, we must ensure that we fulfil the criteria. Before commencing on developing a reflection, always ensure that you fully understand the criteria it will be marked against. If we do not do this as our first step, it is possible that our work will not achieve the result we desire. Further to this, in the same way with all skills, your ability to reflect will increase if you practise. If you continuously practise reflecting, it is more likely that the reflection you submit to be marked will achieve a better result than if the reflection that is assessed is your first.

As well as viewing reflection as a process involving formal writing, we also tend to think of it as being something we do after an experience. This does not need to be the case. It is possible to reflect on an experience while we are having it. Reflection in action is of great value in nursing because it enables us to change the outcome of an experience while it is in progress.

While applying mindfulness to your nursing practice is a good strategy, as it brings both self-kindness and increases self-care, it is not the same as reflecting. Mindfulness involves acceptance, reflection involves questioning, and it is by questioning our experiences that we can improve patient care.

When you reflect, especially if your reflection is not being formally marked, use an approach that you enjoy. There are many creative ways to reflect, and reflection does not have to be a solitary activity. If you use your imagination, reflection does not always have to be a task – it can be also be fun.

GOING FURTHER

Jasper, M. (2013) *Beginning Reflective Practice* (2nd edn). Cengage Learning EMEA. This is an excellent book that uses practice-based examples to assist you to understand the concept of reflective practice.

Koshy, K., Limb, C., Gundogan, B., Whitehurst, K. and Jafree, D. (2017) Reflective practice in health care and how to reflect effectively. *International Journal of Surgical Oncology*, 2(6): e20. An interesting article that offers a simple approach to undertaking reflections.

Sketchnoting for reflection. Go to: http://langwitches.org/blog/2015/08/11/sketchnoting-for-reflection/. An example of how sketchnoting was applied to reflective situations.

ANSWERS TO ACTIVITIES

Activity 5.1

1. A further benefit of formal written reflections is that they enable us to make links between theory and practice, which is an important aspect in developing nursing knowledge.
2. I like writing formal reflections and find that they do enable me to learn. I think that the formality of this way of reflecting can constrain my thinking, though. I view a formal written reflection as an appropriate way to officially demonstrate my ability to consider my actions, understand my strengths and weaknesses, and highlight what I need to develop. I don't find this approach helpful when doing short everyday reflections.

(Continued)

Activity 5.2

1.   Elements of a formal written reflection that I think are important to include are:

- Explicitly applies a reflective model or framework.
- Includes a clear, detailed and appropriate description of the experience being reflected on.
- Demonstrates self-awareness.
- Relates relevant theories, concepts and strategies to nursing practice.
- Is well presented.
- Is critical and analytical.
- Supports views discussed with evidence.
- Correct referencing (follows the format required).
- Effective written communication.

2.   See Table 5.2 below.

Table 5.2   Marking criteria of the elements of a formal written reflection

Criteria	Marks available
Explicitly applies a reflective model or framework.	10
Includes a clear, detailed and appropriate description of the experience being reflected on.	10
Demonstrates self-awareness.	15
Relates relevant theories, concepts and strategies to nursing practice.	10
Is well presented.	5
Is critical and analytical.	25
Supports views discussed with evidence.	10
Correct referencing (follows the format required).	5
Effective written communication.	10
Total	100

You will see in my criteria that I have allocated the most marks to the reflection being critical and analytical. This would be expected during the final year of a nursing programme or of a registered nurse. During the first and second years of a nursing programme, the criteria would be similar, but the focus on critical and analytical writing would be less.

Activity 5.3

1.   See Table 5.3 below.

Table 5.3   Marking Angus's reflection

Criteria	Marks available	Marks awarded to Angus
Explicitly applies a reflective model or framework.	10	7
Includes a clear, detailed and appropriate description of the experience being reflected on.	10	6

Criteria	Marks available	Marks awarded to Angus
Demonstrates self-awareness.	15	7
Relates relevant theories, concepts and strategies to nursing practice.	10	3
Is well presented.	5	4
Is critical and analytical.	25	5
Supports views discussed with evidence.	10	2
Correct referencing (follows the format required).	5	2
Effective written communication.	10	6
Total	100	42

2.   Feedback for Angus on his reflection:

This is an interesting reflection, and it is clear that your first day in placement provided you with a great deal of learning.

You have made an attempt to apply Borton's model, which is appropriate for the reflection you have written. You could have improved your application of this model by:

- highlighting in more detail your rationale for choosing this model; you said that it was the easiest to understand, but you need to develop your rationale further;
- outlining the aim of each of the stages (the aim of first stage is to describe the experience, the second stage aims to enable making sense of the experience and the final stage focuses on plans for what to do next) would have provided evidence that you clearly understood the model;
- being more explicit in the final stage as to what your planned future actions are.

You described the experience you are reflecting on, but you needed to make this more detailed and focused. It would have been appropriate to describe the specific incident which made you realise how unconfident you were feeling, rather than talking about the incident in a more general manner.

You demonstrate in your reflection that you are aware of your actions and clearly have some self-awareness. However, if you had written explicitly about it, this aspect would have been improved.

One area where the reflection needs developing is in the consideration of theory and concepts. This is an important aspect of a reflection that you need to include. You do highlight some strategies of how you are going to act in future, but this also needs further development.

The reflection is visually well presented and the material is considered in a logical fashion with links between the sections. Well done!

Being critical and analytical is an area where your reflection needs development. This is a skill which will improve with practice, but make this an area to work on. You also need to develop your ability to support the points you make with appropriate evidence. Use relevant literature, such as research-based journal articles, professional standards and clinical practice guides to do this. In this reflection you only made one reference to *The Code* (NMC, 2018) but there need to be more.

(Continued)

You have referenced *The Code* correctly in the written text, but remember that you must also include a reference list at the end of the reflection.

Your reflection is generally well written and your spelling and grammar are good. The writing style you use is a little 'chatty', though. If you include evidence and be more critical and analytical, this would improve it.

In summary, Angus, you have made a good first attempt at a reflection, and you are clearly starting to develop your skills. Keep practising your reflective writing and make a note of the areas highlighted here for you to develop.

Well done – you should be pleased with what you have achieved in your first reflection.

Activity 5.4

1.   See Table 5.4 below.

Table 5.4   Marking Gail's reflection

Criteria	Marks available	Marks awarded to Gail
Explicitly applies a reflective model or framework.	10	8
Includes a clear, detailed and appropriate description of the experience being reflected on.	10	8
Demonstrates self-awareness.	15	12
Relates relevant theories, concepts and strategies to nursing practice.	10	8
Is well presented.	5	4
Is critical and analytical.	25	19
Supports views discussed with evidence.	10	8
Correct referencing (follows the format required).	5	5
Effective written communication.	10	8
Total	100	80

2.   Feedback for Gail on her reflection:

This is an excellent final reflection and you should be commended on the standard of the work you have produced.

You have clearly applied Borton's reflective model and the reflection progresses effectively through the three stages. To further improve this, there could have been a more extensive rationale to support the choice of Borton's model over others. I would have liked to have known exactly how you felt it suited the reflection. Further to this, an indication of the aim of the stages would have proved your clear understanding of the model.

You have managed the challenge of being asked to reflect on two differing situations by thinking about common 'themes' for reflection from both professional and academic experiences. This could have been further improved by making more explicit links between the issue of time management and prioritisation.

The issue of self-awareness is carefully considered and clearly demonstrated, and the reflection is strong in the application of theory, concepts and strategies throughout.

You have visually presented the work well and the material considered progresses logically. There is a consistently good level of critical consideration of the issues highlighted and the level of analysis is also sound. This could have been further improved by adopting a more interrogative approach to the evidence.

The use of evidence is a further strength of the reflection. There is a good academic writing style throughout, and the reference format is correct in the text and reference list.

In summary, Gail, you have produced an excellent final reflection. You should be very proud of what you have achieved. Keep practising your reflective writing, make a note of the areas highlighted here for your further development.

Very well done.

3. Differences between Gail's and Angus's reflections:

It is evident in Gail's reflection that she has more experience of reflective writing than Angus. If you look at the topics we have covered so far in this textbook, Gail is including them all at a more developed level than Angus. As has already been said, reflection is just the same as any other skill; the more you practise it, the better you get.

Gail is being more critical than Angus in her writing; she is considering a wide range of evidence and relating it to her experience. Angus's work is much more limited in this respect. Again, as we have said, reflection enables us to understand ourselves, and self-awareness is an area where Gail's reflection is stronger than Angus's. The same can also be said about the application of theory; again, Gail is doing this more effectively than Angus. The final major difference is in the writing style. Gail has a more academic writing style than Angus, which again results in a more advanced reflection.

Activity 5.5

1. Charlie is reflecting on action because he is reflecting after the experience has happened and making plans to act differently in the future.
2. Billy is reflecting in action because he is reflecting while an experience happens and changing his actions at that time.

GLOSSARY

cognitive   Relating to thought processes.

concept   An idea or guiding principle.

explicit   Stated clearly and in detail.

intuitive   Known instinctively.

retrospectively   Looking back over things in the past.

REFERENCES

Borton, T. (1970) *Reach, Touch and Teach*. London: Hutchinson.

Johns, C. (2017) *Becoming a Reflective Practitioner*. Oxford: Wiley-Blackwell.

Nursing and Midwifery Council (NMC) (2018) *The Code*. London: NMC.

Schön, D.A. (1991) *The Reflective Practitioner: How Professionals Think in Action*. Aldershot: Ashgate Publishing.

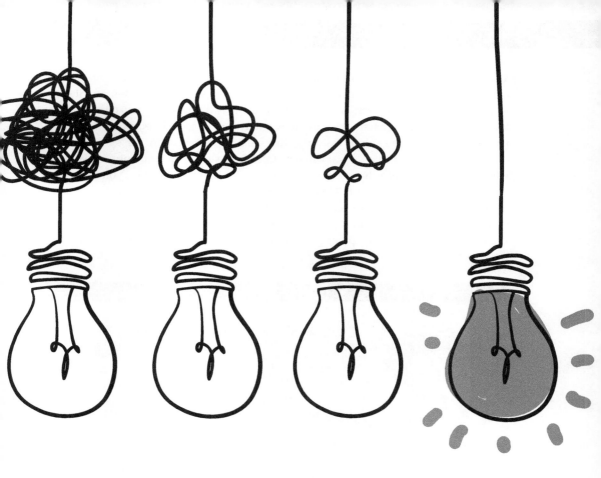

PART B

APPLYING REFLECTION

The second part of the book will enable you to apply reflective practice to your nursing care, appreciate how knowledge can be found in experience and develop an effective action plan based on reflection. We will also consider the role that reflection plays in knowing yourself as a practitioner, and how reflection can assist in ensuring the quality and strategies you can apply to assist you to have time for reflection.

At the start of each chapter you will hear from a registered nurse and nursing student, who are very likely to be sharing the challenges and asking the questions you are, as you continue your journey towards 'being reflective'.

Before you start to read the chapters in this part, however, I would like to introduce you to Florence Kidogo, who is going to share her thoughts and her first reflection for revalidation with you. As we progress through this part of the book, we will refer back to Florence's reflection.

CASE STUDY

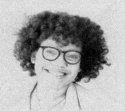

FLORENCE KIDOGO, REGISTERED NURSE, ADULT FIELD

Florence is 35 years old and qualified as an adult nurse two years ago. Prior to commencing nursing, Florence worked part-time as a health care assistant (HCA), mainly on night shifts. Once her two children were at school, she decided that it was time for her to go to university to become a nurse.

To help manage the issues of shifts and childcare, Florence commenced a job in the community as soon as she registered and she is now a community nurse working in a rural area.

As it is two years since Florence registered, she needs to write five reflections in time for her revalidation (NMC, 2016), within the next six to ten months. Florence knows that they can be about continuous professional development, related to feedback she has received about her practice, or about a professional experience or event. She knows, too, that there is a template she must use from the NMC, which she assumes will be helpful. However, although she has written plenty of reflections as a student, it was never one of her strengths and she is worried about having to write them again for revalidation.

Florence's line manager, Anna, knowing that Florence is anxious about the revalidation reflections, suggested that she writes a reflection about her patient, Margaret, who is at the end of her life.

HELLO, FLORENCE KIDOGO HERE!

My line manager has suggested that I write a reflection about my patient, Margaret, as my first reflection for revalidation. I know that there is a template for reflection on the NMC website (NMC, 2016), but I think I'm going to use the model of 'What?, So what? Now what?' by Borton (1970), as I remember from my student days that this is a straightforward model to use and I can present it under the headings that the NMC (2016) uses, which are:

'What was the nature of . . . ' (so this would be the 'What?')

'What did you learn from . . . ' (so this would be the 'So what?')

'How did you change or improve your practice as a result?' (so this would be the 'Now what?').

The last section on the NMC framework asks how the reflection is relevant to the NMC *Code*, and I think this will be quite easy to also fit into the 'Now what?'

I'm going to reflect on looking after Margaret, as I have been upset nursing her. She is at the end of her life and has been in a lot of pain, which has been very distressing both for Margaret and her family. I've found it difficult to help Margaret manage her pain. I think if I reflect on this situation, it might help me to learn from it for the future, and it will also allow me to write my first revalidation reflection!

FLORENCE'S REFLECTION

WHAT?

I have been looking after Margaret ever since I started working as a community nurse. She had leg ulcers, so I was regularly visiting her to dress them. In the last six months, she has developed bone **metastases**, secondary to the breast cancer that had been treated for many years ago. She is now at the end of her life and my job is to make sure she is as comfortable as possible, and do everything possible for her and her family.

The situation has been very difficult. Margaret is in a lot of pain and the family are distressed, both by Margaret's pain and the thought of imminently losing her. I am also sad, as I know Margaret and her family very well, having looked after her for two years.

SO WHAT?

I am very fond of Margaret and her family, and because of this I think I found it difficult to be objective about her care, particularly related to pain management. I tried to offer many alternatives – e.g. regular **oramorph**, then **bupenorphine** patches of increasing strength (NICE, 2012), but somehow I didn't want to discuss with the doctor the prescription of **anticipatory medicines** or a **syringe driver** (NICE, 2015). Doing this signified to me that we were at the end, and this was distressing for me. I was also worried about the complexities of drawing up the different medications within a syringe driver, as I have not had to administer one many times before. I was nervous about the process. Eventually, a syringe driver was prescribed, Margaret's pain and distress were controlled, and her family and I also became less distressed.

NOW WHAT?

I need to put my emotions relating to the feelings that I have for a person and their family to one side, and try to be totally rational in relation to providing care, particularly relating to pain relief and end-of-life care. In my head, a syringe driver signified the end and a last resort, but it is an important consideration for patients in significant pain whether towards the end of life or earlier. I also found that drawing up a syringe driver is not as difficult as I had anticipated, and I will have more confidence in the future when preparing syringe drivers.

This reflection is relevant to many elements within *The Code* (NMC, 2018), such as 'Prioritising People', and it also relates specifically to 20.6, which states: 'stay

(Continued)

objective and have clear professional boundaries at all times with people in your care (including those who have been in your care in the past), their families and carers'.

FLORENCE'S THOUGHTS FOLLOWING HER REFLECTION

I have to admit that when Anna first suggested writing the reflection about Margaret I wasn't very keen, but it was actually a lot easier than I thought it would be. Using Borton's framework (1970) really helped, and it has really made me realise that I was letting my feelings about syringe drivers stop me from using one because I believed that syringe drivers mean 'the end', and I was worried about the complexity of drawing up the medication for a syringe driver. I also researched the use of pain relief for cancer pain and end-of-life care, which was also useful.

Reflecting has allowed me to recognise that I was very emotionally involved with the family and that it is important to step back, remain compassionate, but detached as well, so that I can make the right decisions in everyone's best interests. It has also made me realise that drawing up medication for a syringe driver is not as hard as I thought it was.

Finally, I also now have a first reflection for revalidation written, which is great, and I don't feel so worried about writing four more. Hooray!

GLOSSARY

anticipatory medicines   Medicines prescribed in advance to make sure that a patient being nursed at home has access to medicines they will need if they develop distressing symptoms.

buprenorphine   A drug used to treat pain.

metastases   Malignant growths that develop at a distance from the primary site of a cancer.

oramorph   A drug in a liquid form used as a pain killer.

syringe driver   A small infusion pump used to administer small amounts of fluid to a patient.

REFERENCES

Borton, T. (1970) *Reach, Touch and Teach*. London: Hutchinson.

National Institute for Health and Care Excellence (NICE) (2012) Palliative care for adults: strong opioids for pain relief CG140. Available at: www.nice.org.uk/guidance/cg140/chapter/introduction (accessed 23 August 2020).

NICE (2015) Care of dying adults in the last days of life, NG31. Available at: www.nice.org.uk/guidance/ng31/chapter/Recommendations (accessed 23 August 2020).

Nursing and Midwifery Council (NMC) (2016) Revalidation/What you need to do. Written reflective accounts. Available at: http://revalidation.nmc.org.uk/what-you-need-to-do/written-reflective-accounts/index.html (accessed 23 August 2020).

NMC (2018) *The Code*. London: NMC.

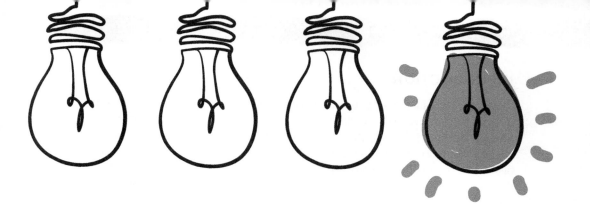

IMPROVING CARE THROUGH REFLECTION

6

CATHERINE DELVES-YATES AND REBEKAH HILL

> " I hate feeling so unconfident about doing the drug round. There are so many liquids and tablets, I'm never going to learn them all. What if I harm a patient by making a drug error? I feel very frightened about this.
>
> **Sheena Marsh, nursing student, learning disability field** "

> " I can really see the value of reflection on a personal level and I use it to make sure that I deliver the best care I can. I am just uncertain of how reflection can be used on a wider scale in order to improve the quality of patient care.
>
> **Humphrey Leachat, registered nurse, adult field** "

INTRODUCTION

Improving the patient care you deliver is a professional responsibility and reflection is an excellent way to ensure that improvements are made as part of your everyday practice. The NMC (2018) identifies that reflection is central to achieving and maintaining good standards, underlining the important role it plays in improving patient care. It is the responsibility of all nurses to become reflective practitioners, improving care by asking questions, not taking any actions for granted, and being enquiring in all you do. Reflection on our actions should become a process we adopt continuously in order to improve our nursing practice, knowledge and skills. This includes reflecting on our own practice and that of others.

In our everyday personal life it would be unusual if we did not think about our day, question something that had been said or had happened, and think about what we might do differently, or the same, next time. We use the same processes when we reflect professionally, the only difference being that we use evidence to underpin what we intend to do in future and formulate a plan to ensure that the care we provide patients with is the best we can deliver. Sheena and Humphrey, who we heard from at the start of the chapter, raise interesting issues. Sheena is worried about her ability to deliver effective care, and although Humphrey is using reflection to ensure that he provides the best care, he isn't sure how reflection can ensure the quality of patient care. Within this chapter we will consider exactly how reflection can aid them both.

─────────────── CHAPTER AIMS ───────────────

This chapter will enable you to:

- understand the differences and similarities between knowledge and experience;
- appreciate how knowledge can be found in experience and identify how you can apply this to your practice;
- consider the importance of being able to reflect while you are 'in action';
- identify strategies that will assist you to have time for reflection;
- develop an effective action plan based on a reflection;
- recognise the role of reflection in ensuring quality.

WHAT ARE KNOWLEDGE AND EXPERIENCE?

ACTIVITY 6.1

Before reading any further, find a definition for the following words:

knowledge;

experience.

Check the activity answers at the end of the chapter to see if the definitions we found were similar.

If we think about the generally accepted definitions of 'knowledge' and 'experience', they can both seem very similar. Knowledge can be thought of as the information and skills gained through education or experience. Similarly, experience can be thought of as the knowledge and skill gained by a period of practical involvement in a specific situation. In fact, the two words are often used in each other's definition, which does little to help us to differentiate between them.

However, if we look in detail at the definitions of knowledge and experience, it becomes clear that:

- knowledge emphasises theory and gaining information or ideas;
- experience involves practice and applying knowledge over a period of time in order to reinforce the understanding of a subject or action.

Viewing 'knowledge' and 'experience' in this way makes it possible to appreciate a difference. The knowledge we gain from being taught provides the foundation for our experience. Although we can increase our knowledge about a subject or action through experience, we cannot obtain experience through being taught. Experience only comes with time and practice.

So, although there are differences in the meaning and purpose of knowledge and experience, it is fair to say that they are closely related. In fact, they work best when used together. When knowledge and experience are applied in combination, they provide us with wisdom – the ability to think and act using knowledge and experience in addition to common sense, understanding and insight. It is actually wisdom that enables us to improve patient care.

THINKING ABOUT EXPERIENCE

In Chapter 1 we discussed that experience is a word that can be used in three different ways. If you refer back to Figure 1.3 on page 11, you can remind yourself of this discussion. As we said, while the word 'experience' can be used as both a noun and a verb, in nursing we most frequently use it to refer to the knowledge and skills (or wisdom) we gain through being involved in a specific situation.

If we think further about the experience gained through being involved in a situation, it becomes clear that there are two kinds of experience: our own and that of others. Although it is highly valuable, gaining our own experience can be a slow and sometimes laboured process – for example, it may take us many years of practice to master a skill. It is, however, possible to benefit more quickly from the experience gained by others. Plus, we can use it as a readily available 'set of instructions' to speed up our learning. We just need to recognise that this type of experience exists and that we can use it as a resource.

HOW CAN KNOWLEDGE BE FOUND IN EXPERIENCE?

You may be aware of the saying 'Experience is the best teacher'. The earliest version of this saying was by Julius Caesar (100–44BCE), the Roman politician, military general and historian who wrote 'Experience is the teacher of all things'. While experience can teach us important lessons – for example, not to touch a hot pan because it will burn us – it is not always a reliable teacher. If, for example, we keep taking risks and repeatedly have near misses from which we escape unscathed, experience could teach us the wrong lesson. What we would learn is that it is fine to take a risk because all will be well. However, such a strategy is likely to eventually end in disaster.

So, while we need to regard experience with an element of caution, it is the foundation for our learning. In order to improve your patient care, you need to consider your experience, using knowledge, information and evidence to critically review the experience, discover what you have learnt and identify what you need to change, as Figure 6.1 shows.

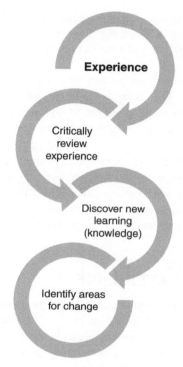

Figure 6.1   Using experience to improve patient care

ACTIVITY 6.2

- Review Figure 6.1 and consider what has been discussed in previous chapters.
- Does Figure 6.1 remind you of anything?

Check the activity answers at the end of the chapter to see if our thoughts are similar.

HOW CAN WE DERIVE USEFUL KNOWLEDGE FROM EXPERIENCE?

It is possible to convert experience into knowledge using reflection. If we review Figure 6.1, the steps identified are the same as those highlighted within many reflective models. If we use relevant evidence to help us to consider our experience, it is possible to discover new learning (or knowledge) and identify ways in which we can improve care. In this way, knowledge can be derived from experience – this is what we referred to as wisdom at the start of the chapter.

Reflection is a process of gradual self-awareness, **critical appraisal** and transformation (Middleton, 2017). Reflection has to be performed intentionally, requires great effort and is not easy to do. Like any exercise, however, if you practise you can increase your ability. The more you reflect on your experiences, the quicker you will learn, and the more your nursing practice will improve.

HOW DO I DERIVE KNOWLEDGE FROM MY EXPERIENCE?

As we have already mentioned, reflection is the key to deriving knowledge from your experience. In fact, this is exactly what you have been doing in all of the reflections you have already undertaken. Although there are many different models of reflection, most can be related to Kolb's (1984) **Experiential** Learning Theory. Kolb (1984, p. 38) identifies that, 'learning is the process whereby knowledge is created through the transformation of experience'. So, Kolb is telling us that we learn by reflecting on what we do.

ACTIVITY 6.3

- Using an online search engine or a library search tool, find a diagram showing the four stages of Kolb's (1984) experiential learning theory.
- Keep this diagram in mind as you read through the next section of this chapter.

There is no definitive answer for this activity.

Kolb's (1984) experiential learning theory involves a cycle of four stages:

1.   Concrete experience.
2.   Reflective observation.
3.   Abstract **conceptualisation**.
4.   Active experimentation.

What Kolb outlines is, for learning to occur, an individual progresses through a cycle of having an experience, reflecting on that experience, learning from the experience and then applying what has been learnt.

If you consider this and look at Figure 6.1, you will find that the same actions are being described, just using slightly different words. In fact, in respect of the words used by Kolb, we need to think professionally about what he refers to as 'active experimentation'. As professionals, we would never 'experiment' in any way while delivering care. As the NMC (2018) states, we must deliver care at all times, which we know is in a patient's best interest. What is being referred to in Kolb's 'active experimentation' stage is the delivery of care, which is based on the 'updated' wisdom (knowledge and experience) we have gained from our reflection. At all times, the care we deliver must be based on contemporary and trustworthy knowledge, so when we undertake an action we know exactly what the outcome will be (unlike an experiment, when the outcome is uncertain).

When we subject our experiences to reflection, it is possible to find knowledge in our experience. In addition to this, we can write down our experiences and share them with others, so not only do we learn from our experience, but others can too. We can also read the experiences of others, so, as we mentioned earlier in the chapter, we can learn from others. In this way, the wisdom we all generate is shared.

Often, you will find that experiences nurses have, which they then reflect on and decide that they wish to investigate further, become the focus of a research project. This is something we will consider in more detail later in the chapter, but by doing this it is possible for experience, when reflected on, to generate further wisdom to improve nursing care and become a useful resource.

ACTIVITY 6.4

Read the Florence Kidogo case study in Part B.

- What knowledge has Florence gained from her experience of caring for Margaret?

Check the activity answers at the end of the chapter to see if our thoughts are similar.

In her reflection on caring for Margaret, Florence Kidogo chose to use Borton's reflective framework. Borton (1970) cleverly uses just three short questions to get us to think critically about our experience.

If we consider what Florence says, she most certainly has gained knowledge from her experience, both about herself and about caring for a patient. She is developing her wisdom, and by reading her reflection we are also able to learn from it. Florence can now apply what she has learnt to her practice in order to ensure that she delivers the best care possible.

One of the most important aspects of reflection is that it encourages our thinking and learning. Remember to use reflection to identify what has gone well, as well as pondering over events that did not turn out how you wished. Think about, for example, the patient whose questions you were able to answer, the procedure you performed with accuracy and skill. Use these events to celebrate that you kept up to date with relevant evidence and guidance. Lessons can always be learned from what went wrong, but equally they can be learned from what went right; you just need to ask 'why?' and 'how?'.

Reflection can be used to improve care in a number of ways: it aids the integration of theory and practice, and also enhances learning from experience. Reflection increases self-awareness and insight into your behaviour and responses, enabling you to analyse your attitudes and relationships. All these factors enable you to learn from your experiences.

REFLECTION IN ACTION

If we think about Florence Kidogo's reflection, what Florence is doing is reflecting on her actions after they have happened. This, as we have said, is useful and will enable her, in future, to ensure that in a similar situation she can apply what she has learnt. Reflection, however, can be used more immediately than this if we reflect while we are in action. This is something we discussed in Chapter 5, and if Florence had been able to act in this way she could have improved the care she was offering to Margaret at the time, rather than have to wait to apply her learning to another patient.

As Johns (2017) highlights, we need to develop a constant state of mindfulness in our practice, so we are constantly being reflective. If we refer to material we considered in Chapter 1 and in particular look at Figure 1.1 on page 8, we can see how reflection really is like an onion, so to make it as useful as possible, we need to work our way through each of the layers.

If we consider Florence's actions, she is at the 'reflection on experience' layer. Florence has considered a previous experience and taken into account the new knowledge gained from this. To develop her reflective skills, she now needs to start considering what is happening as the experience occurs and, in real time, modify her actions based on the knowledge she is gaining. This is reflection in action (Schön, 1983). When Florence is caring for patients, she needs to start to 'think on her feet', carefully considering what her next actions should be and acting on this knowledge immediately. This brings the benefit of having more control over a situation. By taking action at the time, Florence can ensure that the care she is delivering at that moment is the best possible, rather than waiting until after the event and then realising that she could have acted differently. So, by moving to the 'reflection in action' layer of the onion, it is possible to use reflection as a tool to ensure that you deliver the best possible care.

This is a big step to take. It is a skill that needs work to develop the ability to be critical of your own actions as you undertake them and be constantly attuned to the responses of others. The key to this is being critical and ensuring that you have sound evidence to challenge your practice and that of others. Reflection is a highly beneficial tool if it is used to improve practice, but it has no value if it validates poor practice by ignoring evidence. Without critical thought, outdated attitudes or practices can be left unchallenged. Effective critical reflection is that which challenges practice, results in changes and enables you to use experience to improve care. Reflection is an important way to develop practice because it helps you make sense of experience, seek alternatives and improvements, all based on sound evidence.

If we think back to the issues raised by Sheena and Humphrey at the start of this chapter, it is now possible to answer some of their questions. If Sheena uses both reflection on action and reflection in action, she can develop her knowledge of medications and their administration to ensure that her actions are safe at all times. Sheena is correct: there are numerous medications to learn about, and even the most experienced nurses will tell you that this is a topic they continue to study. Sheena can, however, reflect (on action) on her feelings of fear and adopt a reflect (in action) safe approach to medications administration to ensure that she does not give a patient any drug without being certain that it is correct.

Humphrey already understands how reflection can assist him to improve his individual practice, which of course also does have a wider impact as this will improve the quality of care delivered to the patients he cares for. Humphrey will also be acting as a role model for his colleagues, which will have a positive impact on the entire area. We will return to Humphrey's questions and the topic of reflection as a quality improvement tool later in this chapter.

CREATING TIME TO REFLECT

While the benefits of reflection are clear, time, or lack of it, is a potential barrier. Effective reflection takes time and effort, so we need to find ways to make this less **onerous**. Like any exercise, practice makes you quicker. Some strategies that nurses use to integrate reflection into their everyday life and professional practice are:

- Reflect on your day during your journey home, considering what went well and what could have been improved.
- Keep a reflective diary or just keep a written record of the outcome of your reflections.
- Join (or start) a reflection group in your clinical area.
- Engage in clinical supervision or find a mentor.

If you are **innovative**, it is possible to find more ways to reflect without it being too time-consuming. If you consistently practise reflection, you will become engaged in a constant process of self-education, improving your practice and continually developing your skills. Remember, your experience can be used to benefit others, so make a written record of your reflections, highlighting what you have learnt and think about how you can share this wisdom. You could do this in a formal manner, publishing your reflection in a nursing journal, for example, or in a less formal way by sharing your reflection with your colleagues or peers. You may find that you want to expand your learning from your reflections even further and use them to develop a **quality improvement proposal** or a research project. We will discuss this further later in this chapter.

Always remember that reflection is far too valuable a tool to be seen only as a task you complete for assignments or revalidation. Reflection is something you can adapt to the needs of your patients, yourself and your practice area to ensure that maximum benefit is gained.

HOW REFLECTION CAN BE ACTED ON

Reflection should be used to develop your knowledge in nursing practice and improve your care. The key to successful reflection is the completion of a learning cycle (Kolb, 1984), ensuring that you create an action plan as a result of your learning from reflection. In this way, you will also apply what you have learnt to your nursing care.

One of the many benefits of reflection is that it will help you to improve your self-awareness, from which you will constantly learn. Reflection also enables you to take personal responsibility for your actions and improvements, and importantly, it engages you in your own development.

As we have already discussed, reflecting on practice is an essential attribute of competent nurses. If the challenges facing nurses on a daily basis are considered – the need to constantly cope with uncertainty, frequent change and a high demand for services – it is hardly surprising that stress, burnout and high attrition rates are an ongoing concern. Using reflective practice as a way to improve the mindfulness of the practitioners, as well as the quality of the care they deliver, is a helpful strategy to address this.

ACTIVITY 6.5

Read Florence Kidogo's reflection in Part B.

- Write an action plan for Florence to enable her to implement the learning she has gained from her reflection.

Check the activity answers at the end of the chapter to see if our thoughts are similar.

THE ROLE OF REFLECTION IN ENSURING QUALITY

Being a reflective practitioner means that you are constantly enquiring, questioning assumptions, looking for answers to puzzles or questions from your observations, dilemmas and critical incidents, and transforming these into action to develop professional expertise. The responsibility that nurses have for providing care goes hand in hand with the responsibility to ensure its quality, and applying a critical reflective approach can play an important role in ensuring this.

Improving quality is a professional responsibility; using reflection will ensure that quality is part of your everyday practice. Reflective practice is a way of ensuring that quality care is delivered and quality decisions are made (Stonehouse, 2015). There are many ways to monitor and improve quality, such as clinical audit, performance benchmarking, patient feedback, process maps and cause-and-effect diagrams, and in addition to all this, personal reflection has much to offer as an approach to ensure quality (Johns, 2017). Indeed, evaluation of the quality of your work, and that of others, is a requirement of the NMC *Code* (2018).

Reflection is essential in order to maintain standards of care; it is crucial to detect and increase awareness of care erosion. Self-awareness and self-correction are vital qualities in nurses. By knowing yourself, you will recognise the discomfort felt when there is an inconsistency between care standards in practice and those you value; when there is **dissonance** between what you experience and what you expect, you must act. For reflections to improve care, they have to be critical in nature and the emphasis has to be on taking action as a result of learning. Reflection improves care by developing understanding, from which you can bring about improvements and change, which are often called 'quality improvements'.

ACTIVITY 6.6

The following link will take you to a range of quality improvement projects that were developed because of the realisation that the current care being delivered could be better:

www.health.org.uk/search/basic_page_sub_type/48/basic_page_sub_type/55?
textsearch=improvement%20projects&sort_by=created&sort_order=DESC

(Continued)

Read about one of the projects you find interesting.

- Considering how care was developed in the quality improvement project you read, suggest an area of care that Florence highlights in her reflection in Part B, which could be the focus of a quality improvement proposal.

Check the activity answers at the end of the chapter to see if our thoughts are similar.

If we consider Humphrey's question at the start of the chapter again, at both an individual and organisational level, the impact of reflective practice should be a process of continual questioning of assumptions and accepted ways of doing things. This will lead to transformation and quality improvement on an ongoing basis. The potential benefits of this are immense – better decision making, better care, increased staff well-being and engagement, and, perhaps also, fewer incidents and complaints.

CONCLUSION

Nurses have a responsibility to become reflective practitioners and improve practice by asking questions and not taking their actions for granted (NMC, 2018). Reflecting on practice is an essential attribute of competent nurses. We learn by reflecting on what we do; one of the most important things about reflection is that it encourages our thinking and learning.

Reflecting on our actions enables us to convert experience into knowledge, and applying knowledge in combination with experience provides us with wisdom. The best way to view this wisdom is as the ability to think and act using knowledge and experience in addition to common sense, understanding and insight. It is wisdom that enables us to improve patient care.

Reflection is far too valuable a tool to be seen only as a task you complete for assignments or revalidation. Reflection is something you can adapt to the needs of your patients, yourself and your practice area to ensure that maximum benefit is gained. For reflections to improve care, however, they have to be critical in nature and the emphasis has to be on taking action as a result of learning.

────────────────── GOING FURTHER ──────────────────

Johns, C. (2017) *Becoming a Reflective Practitioner*. Chichester: Wiley-Blackwell. Using a contemporary approach, this book presents a variety of reflective extracts that will challenge you to question your own practice.

Middleton, R. (2017) Critical reflection: the struggle of a practice developer. *International Practice Development Journal*, 7(1): 4. This article seeks to explore why reflection is difficult for some, sharing personal stories of a practice developer's experiences of wrestling with reflective models and learning to reflect in a meaningful way.

Improving the quality of care. Go to: www.hcpc-uk.org/news-and-events/news/2019/hcpc-unites-with-health-regulators-to-issue-joint-statement-in-support-reflective-practice-across-healthcare/. An interesting web-link in which the Health and Care Professions Council identifies that reflective practice improves the quality of care.

ANSWERS TO ACTIVITIES

Activity 6.1

1. Knowledge can be defined as the facts, information and skills acquired by a person through experience or education; the theoretical or practical understanding of a subject. Knowledge is what is known in a particular field or in total – facts and information – and is 'true', justified belief, certain understanding, as opposed to opinion.
2. Experience can be defined as practical contact with and observation of facts or events. It is the knowledge or skill acquired by experience over a period of time, especially that gained in a particular profession by someone at work. It can also be an event or occurrence that leaves an impression on someone.

Activity 6.2

Figure 6.1 reminds me of a reflective model. If you consider the steps it identifies, they are exactly the same as those highlighted within many reflective models.

Activity 6.4

From reflecting on her experience of caring for Margaret, Florence has gained knowledge both about herself and about pain management for patients when they are at the end of life.

Florence identified that she found it difficult to be objective about the care she was delivering to Margaret, and that she found it distressing to view Margaret as being at the end of her life. This is an important realisation, as while Florence needs to be compassionate in her care for Margaret and her family, she needs to approach this in a fashion that ensures that the best care is delivered at all times and not influenced by Florence feeling unable to cope with an issue.

Florence has also learnt about a form of effective pain management for patients who are at the end of their lives and gained practical skills in managing the method of delivering this.

Activity 6.5

When writing an action plan to follow Florence's reflection, I would identify what was needed (the objective to be achieved), how it could be achieved (the plan) and a date for when it should be achieved by, as below. See Chapter 7 for more details on how to write a SMARTER action plan.

(Continued)

Table 6.1   An action plan following Florence's reflection on caring for a patient who is at the end of life

Objective to be achieved	Plan	To be achieved in	Achieved?
Increase my knowledge of the way to manage pain for patients who are at end of life.	Contact specialist nurse at local Trust and ask them to: 1. suggest some reading to develop my knowledge; 2. identify a study day which will improve my knowledge; 3. arrange to spend two shifts working with the specialist nurse to develop my practical skills.	8 weeks' time	Yes/no Further action needed?
Increase my ability to offer effective and compassionate care while remaining objective.	1. Discuss this with my manager and find out how she manages in similar situations. 2. Discuss this with the specialist nurse and find out how they manage in similar situations. 3. Ask my manager to arrange for me to have an experienced nurse as a mentor I can meet with on a regular basis to discuss this. 4. Complete a literature search focusing on objectivity in nursing care to find out how to remain objective while being compassionate.	4 months' time	Yes/no Further action needed?

There is a considerable amount of work for Florence to do in completing this action plan, so although dates have been identified for when the activity should be completed, there is also the option to identify further actions. This is especially important when considering an issue such as Florence's need to develop her ability to remain objective. Even though a four-month deadline has been set, it is likely that this would become an 'ongoing' aspect of Florence's development.

Activity 6.6

Considering Florence's experience in trying to manage Margaret's pain effectively, it would have been helpful if she had a research-based 'tool' to refer to, which would offer guidance as to appropriate medications when Margaret's pain was not being managed effectively. If Florence had a tool to guide her actions, this could help to take the pressure away from her and the feeling that she was making the decision that Margaret was 'near the end'. A good quality improvement for Florence to propose following this experience would be one that identified, implemented and evaluated the use of such a tool.

GLOSSARY

critical appraisal A systematic approach used to identify strengths and weaknesses.

conceptualisation Forming an idea.

dissonance Lack of agreement.

experiential Involving or based on experience and observation.

innovative Introducing new, original and creative ideas.

onerous Involving a great deal of effort or difficulty.

quality improvement proposal A carefully considered and planned approach to improve the quality of care.

REFERENCES

Borton, T. (1970) *Reach, Touch and Teach*. London: Hutchinson.

Johns, C. (2017) *Becoming a Reflective Practitioner*. Chichester: Wiley-Blackwell.

Kolb, D. (1984) *Experiential Learning: Experience as the Source of Learning and Development* (Vol. 1). Englewood Cliffs, NJ: Prentice-Hall.

Middleton, R. (2017) Critical reflection: the struggle of a practice developer. *International Practice Development Journal*, 7(1): 4.

Nursing and Midwifery Council (NMC) (2018) *The Code*. London: NMC.

Schön, D. (1983) *The Reflective Practitioner: How Professionals Think in Action*. London: Temple Smith.

Stonehouse, D. (2015) Reflective practice: ensuring quality care. *British Journal of Healthcare Management*, 21(5): 237–40.

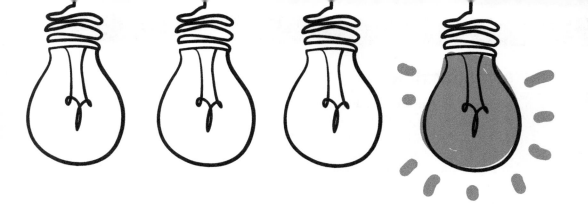

IMPROVING PRACTICE THROUGH REFLECTION

7

CORAL DRANE

> I am writing a reflection focusing on 'opportunistic learning', a 'critical incident' and my 'strengths and weaknesses'. I find it difficult as we have to reflect on the same things for each placement, so it is hard to be original each time. It is also tricky to think of different models to use.
>
> **Sam Valence, nursing student, adult field**

> One of my patients died unexpectedly in the night. Did I miss something? Was it my fault? I am really upset. I think writing a reflection to work out if I could have done anything differently last night might help and enable me to know how to manage similar situations in the future.
>
> **Izzy French, registered nurse, adult field**

INTRODUCTION

Reflection on patient care, as we saw in the previous chapter, is important. In this chapter we will explore in detail the importance of knowing yourself as a practitioner, the role that reflection plays in this, and how this knowledge enables the development of practice on a daily basis.

This chapter will start by analysing how strengths and weaknesses, or limitations, relating to practice can be acknowledged, strengths maximised and weaknesses developed. We will draw on the experience of Florence Kidogo, who we met in Part B, and Sam and Izzy, who we heard from at the start of the chapter, as the chapter unfolds.

Moving on from strengths and weaknesses, we will explore how beliefs and values impact on care, and how knowledge of these, through reflection, supports the development of practice. We will then examine learning styles, as knowledge of how we learn can be used to highlight how best to improve practice.

Finally, we will draw all these elements together and consider how reflection allows us to know ourselves as practitioners and therefore improve our practice.

─────────────── CHAPTER AIMS ───────────────

This chapter will enable you to:

- understand why it is important to acknowledge strengths, weaknesses and limitations in practice;
- appreciate how reflection can maximise strengths and develop weaknesses or limitations;
- know why knowledge of beliefs and values is useful in the development of practice;
- realise how learning styles can be used to improve practice;
- recognise the role of reflection in knowing yourself as a practitioner.

FINDING YOUR STRENGTHS AND LIMITATIONS

Strengths (S) and weaknesses (W) are often analysed in conjunction with opportunities (O) and threats (T) in the form of SWOT analysis. This type of analysis was originally developed in America the 1950–60s and was intended for use in business, but it can also be a useful tool in nursing. The term 'weaknesses' can have negative connotations, so it is more appropriate to use the word 'limitations' instead. Thus, the SWOT analysis becomes a 'SLOT' analysis. Within this section we will focus on how strengths and limitations can be determined, as these tend to be **internally driven**, and therefore relate to knowledge of yourself. Opportunities and threats are often external to ourselves and therefore less controllable, so will not be considered, although it is, of course, equally important to be aware of them.

How can you find out your strengths and limitations, and hence your development needs? It can be difficult to acknowledge what we are good at, or not so good at, but as nurses it is important to find a way to do this so that we increase our self-awareness. Pearce (2007) emphasises that the key to a good SLOT analysis is to be realistic and honest about our strengths. If you struggle to do this, listing your **attributes** can help, as these are likely to underpin your strengths.

To do this, think about your attributes based on your experiences. Let your mind relax and ask yourself the following questions:

- What do I know that I am good at?
- What do I feel confident doing?
- What do I do that makes me feel good?
- What are my best attributes?
- How do I know I am good at/confident at something?
- What positive feedback have I had about something so that I know it is one of my strengths?

Similarly, to determine limitations, the opposite questions can be asked:

- What do I do that I recognise I am not as good at as I would like to be?
- What do I worry about doing?
- What doesn't make me feel good?
- What are my least good attributes?
- How do I know that I am not as strong at these things?

ACTIVITY 7.1

Before reading further, consider the questions above and list your attributes, strengths and limitations.

- Now devise a complete 'SLOT' analysis (strengths, limitations, opportunities, threats) related to your practice or a specific area of your practice.

There is no definitive answer for this activity as it is personal to you, but you could discuss what you have written with a colleague, your practice supervisor or university lecturer.

From the questions we asked in order to identify your attributes, it is clear that feedback from colleagues, patients, friends and family can all help in terms of recognition strengths and limitations. There are many frameworks that can assist you to do this, but two that are particularly helpful are the Johari window (Luft, 1969) and Brookfield's lenses (Brookfield, 1998).

The Johari window was developed by psychologists Joseph Luft and Harry Ingram in 1955 through their work on group dynamics. As shown in Table 7.1, they identified that for every person there are four 'windows' of the self:

1. 'Open' area, known to self and known to others.
2. 'Hidden' area, known to self but hidden from others.
3. 'Blind' area, known to others, but unknown to the self.
4. 'Unknown' area, unknown to self and also unknown to others.

Table 7.1   The Johari window

	Known to self	Unknown to self
Known to others	Open area	Blind area (this becomes smaller after feedback from others).
Unknown to others	Hidden area (this becomes smaller as we share our hidden thoughts or abilities with others).	Unknown area (skills/thoughts unknown and untested by an individual, so unknown to self and to others).

Source: Adapted from Luft (1969)

As we become increasingly self-aware, through feedback from others who recognise our strengths and limitations when we are not able to, our 'blind' area becomes smaller, and so we develop understanding of ourselves. Similarly, we are able to enlarge our 'open' area and reduce our 'hidden' area by sharing our strengths and limitations with others. While it is likely that we use the Johari window **concept** unconsciously, if we become conscious of it, we can increase knowledge of our strengths and limitations.

Developing further the idea of understanding ourselves though discussion with others, Brookfield's lenses may also be helpful. Brookfield (1998) explored how it is possible to critically reflect through the **notion** of four lenses. In the **context** of nursing practice, the 'learner', as noted below, would be the 'patient'. These lenses are:

1.   Our autobiographical lens (e.g. self-reflection).
2.   The lens of the 'learner' or 'patient' (e.g. considering what patients would think about a particular situation).
3.   The lens of colleagues (e.g. gaining feedback from practice colleagues).
4.   The theoretical lens (e.g. reflection related to evidence/research).

Brookfield's work was based on critical reflection for teachers. However, there are parallels in nursing, and 'putting yourself into another person's shoes' by considering how patients or colleagues might view you is informative. Equally, reflecting on strengths and limitations in relation to relevant theory or the evidence base, as Brookfield suggests, can also assist self-awareness.

ACTIVITY 7.2

Think about Brookfield's four lenses.

•   Write a brief analysis of an element of your practice, using the framework Brookfield identifies.

There is no definitive answer for this activity as it is personal to you, but you could discuss what you have written with a colleague, your practice supervisor or university lecturer.

Thinking about Sam's situation, which he shared at the beginning of the chapter, he could use a SLOT analysis, the Johari window, or Brookfield lenses as frameworks for his reflection. Although not 'reflective models', any of these would provide a logical format and allow him to identify ideas he could use in a reflection on his development needs.

If we think about Izzy's situation, again, as we heard at the start of the chapter, she could have a reflective discussion with a colleague asking for feedback about her night shift, using the Johari window. This would open up her 'blind' area within the context of caring for a deteriorating patient. It would also allow her to share her feelings about the night and open up her 'hidden' area, allowing her to learn from the experience. After a death such as Izzy described, there is enormous value in a 'team hot debrief'. This debrief takes place ideally during the same shift as the critical incident so that all of the people involved are available. This approach enables team reflection and learning. In its simplest format, three questions (Paediatric FOAMed, 2018) are asked:

1. What went well?
2. What did not go well?
3. What can we do differently or what needs to change to improve practice?

From this debrief discussion, it is possible to identify key learning and actions. If this happened in Izzy's situation, she would be able to use learning from it for her reflection and it would help her to recognise that it was not her fault that the patient died.

MAXIMISING YOUR STRENGTHS, REDUCING LIMITATIONS

After completing activities in this chapter so far, you will have used a 'SLOT' analysis, considered Brookfield's lenses, and reflected on feedback from patients and colleagues to identify your strengths and limitations. The next step is to devise an action plan so that you can continue to increase your strengths and set objectives to develop your limitations.

Action plans can take many forms, but whenever possible, the goals you set yourself within the action plan need to be SMARTER. The SMARTER **acronym** has many variations, but the key words are:

Specific	**S**ignificant		
Measurable	**M**eaningful	**M**anageable	
Achievable	**A**ttainable	**A**ction-orientated	**A**greed
Realistic	**R**elevant	**R**easonable	**R**esourced
Time-related	**T**rackable		
Evaluated	**E**thical	**E**ngaging	
Reassessed	**R**evisited	**R**ecordable	**R**eviewed

(Adapted from Brown et al., 2016; Moustafa Leonard and Pakdil, 2016)

SMARTER can be adapted to suit your needs, choosing the word from what is the most appropriate for each element. Often the words used within nursing are likely to be:

Specific, Measurable, Achievable, Realistic, Time-related, Evaluated and Reviewed. Sometimes it is not possible to be completely SMARTER, as the time element may not be controllable. It is, however, important to set yourself targets that are realistic, relevant and achievable; unachievable goals will decrease your self-esteem.

If we think about Sam who we met at the start of the chapter, and further develop his experience, when he reflected on his strengths and limitations using a 'SLOT' analysis, he identified that a limitation for him was delegation. He knew himself that this was a concern, as he felt shy asking older, more experienced colleagues to assist him, or to do things for him if he was busy. He had also received feedback from his practice supervisor that this was something he needed to develop. A SMARTER target for him therefore would be 'to improve delegation to colleagues by the end of your next placement' and the SMARTER details would be:

S   Specific target of improving delegation to colleagues.

M   Measurable by self-assessment and feedback from Sam's supervisor, peers and colleagues.

A   Target of improving delegation is achievable.

R   Target of improving delegation is realistic, relevant and reasonable.

T   Time related – by the end of Sam's placement.

E   Evaluation – at the end of his placement, evaluated through self-reflection and feedback.

R   Review – as part of the ongoing evaluation and at the end of his placement, Sam would need to decide whether the goal was still needed or whether it should be reset or modified in any way.

As well as setting SMARTER targets to improve limitations, it is helpful to break down targets and form an action plan. Table 7.2 shows how Sam did this.

Table 7.2   Sam's action plan

Target/objective	Resources needed/ how will I achieve this target?	Success criteria	Target date
Improve delegation skills.	Practise delegating tasks/ actions to colleagues. Talk to fellow students about how they delegate. Ask for feedback from colleagues and practice supervisor to ascertain progress.	Feel confident to delegate appropriately to colleagues. Receive positive feedback about delegation skills from colleagues, practice supervisor and practice assessor.	By the end of my placement.

ACTIVITY 7.3

- Using your SLOT analysis, and the Brookfield framework completed in Activities 7.1 and 7.2, devise an action plan for your development.

There is no definitive answer for this activity as it is personal to the individual, but you could discuss what you have written with a colleague, your practice supervisor or university lecturer.

HOW CAN FLORENCE KIDOGO DISCOVER HER STRENGTHS AND LIMITATIONS?

As we read in Part B, in her reflection Florence identified that she had a very strong compassionate relationship with Margaret and her family, so that was clearly a strength. Florence also felt that she had not been objective when managing Margaret's pain. She felt that she had allowed her own feelings and worries about the use of syringe drivers to prevent her from using one at an earlier stage. So, we can identify the following.

Florence's strengths:

- Provision of compassionate care.
- Commitment to holistic care involving the family.
- Ability to listen to feedback.

Florence's limitations:

- Difficult to remain objective.
- Worried about managing end-of-life care.
- Worried about using syringe drivers as they signify 'the end' and due to the complexity of setting them up.

An action plan for Florence would be:

Table 7.3 Florence's action plan

Target/objective	Resources needed/ how will I achieve this target?	Success criteria/ reviewing progress	Target or review date
Continue to provide compassionate and holistic care.	Ongoing care of patients in the community. Receive feedback from colleagues, patients and their families. Read relevant nursing articles related to community care.	Continue to feel confident with providing compassionate and holistic care. Ongoing positive feedback from colleagues, patients and families.	Next annual appraisal meeting.

(Continued)

Table 7.3   (Continued)

Target/objective	Resources needed/ how will I achieve this target?	Success criteria/ reviewing progress	Target or review date
Develop more objectivity when caring for patients, especially at the end of life.	Discuss the issues with colleagues to gain their insight. Try to separate myself from the situation and 'look in' on what is happening to assess the way forward.	Become confident in remaining objective when managing complex situations such as end of life. Receive positive feedback from colleagues, patients and families.	By the time of revalidation.
Feel more confident in managing end-of-life care.	Research and find suitable end-of-life care course to attend. Attend end-of-life course. Read relevant nursing articles about end-of-life care. Seek support from colleagues where appropriate.	Increased confidence when managing end-of-life care. Receive positive feedback from colleagues, patients and families.	Attend end-of-life course at earliest available opportunity. Ongoing development of confidence.
Develop skills in management of a syringe driver.	Practise drawing up syringe drivers. Discuss process with colleagues. Research evidence for end-of-life medication.	Feel confident with drawing up and administering syringe drivers. Receive positive feedback from colleague, patients and families. Be able to explain confidently to patients and families what the medication is for.	By the time of revalidation.

So, for both Sam and Florence, devising and achieving an action plan would assist them to develop their limitations and increase their strengths.

IDENTIFYING BELIEFS AND VALUES TO IMPROVE YOUR PRACTICE

In the first part of this chapter we have established the importance of recognising strengths and developing limitations in order to improve practice. We will now consider values and beliefs, and how these can impact on our practice.

To begin, it is useful to consider how we define beliefs and values. The *Oxford Dictionary* (2016a) explains that a belief is:

an acceptance that something exists or is true, especially one without proof; e.g., 'his belief in extraterrestrial life'; 'Trust, faith, or confidence in someone or something'.

The *Oxford Dictionary* (2016b) defines value as:

the regard that something is held to deserve; the importance, worth, or usefulness of something; e.g. 'your support is of great value', *or Principles or standards of behaviour; one's judgment of what is important in life, e.g.,* 'they internalize their parents' rules and values'.

As nurses, we might hold beliefs such as 'I am not very good at writing reflections' (possibly Sam's view) or 'it was my fault that he died' (maybe Izzy's view). Examples of personal values that we might hold, based on the definition above, could be the importance of honesty, integrity, person-centredness and compassion (potentially Florence's values).

It is interesting to consider where the beliefs and values held by Sam, Izzy and Florence originated, and whether they are static or evolve over time. The definition we saw suggests that we internalise our parents' values, and although this likely to be a factor, psychologists suggest that our beliefs and values develop from many other sources too.

Erikson (1902–94) wrote about eight developmental stages of **psychosocial** development. His model suggests that we are influenced throughout our entire lives across eight stages of development, depending on 'crises' that occur. Our personalities develop as a result of these successive crises. Therefore, as we progress through life, we adapt and modify our values and beliefs, although it is likely that the foundation of these originate from childhood.

Bandura (1977) considered that social environment impacts on our learning and that through observation we observe and learn behaviours, values and beliefs by the imitation or 'modelling' of other people with whom we identify. This may be parents, but could also be siblings, peers or people we admire in the media, work or elsewhere. We are likely to identify with individuals for whom we have a high regard – our 'role models'– and are motivated to replicate their behaviours, values and beliefs.

A further element of Bandura's work is related to self-efficacy – which is your belief that you are able to achieve a specific goal. So, a person with a positive self-efficacy for a specified goal is likely to achieve that goal. This is a key concept when considering nurses' or nursing students' belief systems. Self-efficacy is developed from self-evaluation and feedback from a wide variety of sources, with negative self-efficacy being developed due to unconstructive feedback. The lack of self-belief which results from this experience can be difficult to reverse.

Our beliefs and values have origins due to 'nurture' (environmental factors – e.g. our upbringing), but also originate in 'nature' (e.g. our genetic code). Some psychologists believe that our personalities are 'pre-wired' before birth, whereas others, such as Bandura, believe that we are a product of our learned experiences. Whatever the source of our values and beliefs, it is important that we are able to identify them, so we are self-aware in order to develop our practice appropriately. It is also vital to recognise that patients and their loved ones have their own core values and beliefs, and that these need to be acknowledged, respected and considered continuously.

ACTIVITY 7.4

Think about what we have considered and write down three of your core beliefs.

- How do you think they might impact on your practice?

There is no definitive answer for this activity as it is personal to you, but you could discuss what you have written with a colleague, your practice supervisor or university lecturer.

HOW CAN KNOWING BELIEFS AND VALUES UPHOLD PRACTICE?

There are a number of important values we need to uphold in our practice. The core values of NHS England (NHS, 2015) are:

- Respect and dignity.
- Commitment to the quality of care.
- Compassion.
- Improving lives.
- Working together for patients.
- Everyone counts.

Further important values that underpin nursing are the 6Cs (NHS, 2012):

- Compassion
- Communication
- Competence
- Commitment
- Care
- Courage

ACTIVITY 7.5

To help you identify the values you could develop in order to improve your practice, consider each of the NHS values and the 6Cs.

- Think about how evident each of these values are in your practice and give each a scale of 0-3 where:

    0 = not evident in my practice;

    1 = occasionally evident in my practice;

    2 = mostly evident in my practice;

    3 = always evident in my practice.

Any values given a score of 2 or less would be a good focus for development, for which you could devise an action plan, as discussed earlier in the chapter.

There is no definitive answer for this activity as it is personal to you, but you could discuss what you have written with a colleague, your practice supervisor or university lecturer.

Considering beliefs in more detail, we are often not aware of them until they are challenged, or we are asked about our specific view. Beliefs in nursing relate to numerous areas – for example, belief in our own ability (self-efficacy); belief in the correct process – e.g. aseptic non-touch technique; person-centred care, our belief in people – e.g. 'Sister Annie is an excellent role model'; belief in education or the belief in being supportive – and the list continues. A reflection on your beliefs could commence by considering your ideas about beliefs (as suggested in Activity 7.4), listing and exploring them, and then analysing how these beliefs impact on you as a practitioner and how this knowledge can be used to improve your practice – for example, using the case of Izzy who we met at the start of the chapter, she believed that it might have been her fault that a patient died. This is clearly a destructive belief. By considering it objectively – e.g. by reflecting on the patient diagnosis, on her own actions and the actions of others in the team, effectively analysing the experience – Izzy will recognise that the death was not her fault, her belief will be modified and she will use the experience to develop her practice.

USING FLORENCE KIDOGO TO HIGHLIGHT HOW BELIEFS AND VALUES CAN BE IDENTIFIED

If we think about Florence, who we met in Part B, we can identify that some of her values relating to the 6Cs were compassion, care, commitment and courage. She was clearly compassionate, caring and committed when nursing Margaret and had the courage to recognise her need to develop in terms of her objectivity. We can assume that her communication with the family was effective, as she clearly had a good rapport with them. Possibly, her competence in the use of a syringe driver for pain relief and end-of-life care was a limitation, and this is something that Florence recognised in her reflection.

Considering her beliefs, Florence believed that using a syringe driver would signify 'the end', which is not correct. She also believed that preparation of the driver would be difficult, which is inaccurate. Recognising these beliefs helped Florence to develop her practice, so in future she will use a syringe driver at a more appropriate time. Analysing Florence's belief systems further, she believed that she had a good rapport with Margaret and her family, which helped her to deliver compassionate care. Knowledge of this positive belief will allow Florence's confidence to grow and she will be able to continue to develop her compassionate approach.

IDENTIFYING YOUR LEARNING STYLE IN ORDER TO IMPROVE YOUR PRACTICE

Self-awareness has many dimensions. In addition to being aware of professional and personal strengths, development needs, values and beliefs, it is helpful to be aware of your learning style. This can most simply be defined as understanding how we learn best. We all learn differently depending on factors such as motivation, personality, environment, context and experience. To find out how you learn, there are numerous learning style questionnaires. Well-known examples include Honey and Mumford (1992) and Dunn et al.'s (1989) learning styles questionnaire. While there is argument that learning style questionnaires are not sufficiently research-based, they can be helpful to identify your preferred learning styles. This enables you to know yourself and to facilitate the development of strategies to support your learning. It can also be valuable to discover the learning styles of individuals you might be supervising, coaching or teaching.

Some people learn effectively through seeing pictures (**V** – visual), some by listening (**A** – aural), some through reading and writing (**R**), while others through doing something (**K** – **kinaesthetic**). This comprises the VARK learning style inventory (VARK, 2019).

In addition to the way we like to learn, identified by VARK, Honey and Mumford (1992) suggest that there are four types of learner: activist, pragmatist, reflector and theorist.

- Activists jump in and are happy to try things before really finding out about them.
- Pragmatists are practical in their approach to learning.
- Reflectors like to weigh everything up and ponder.
- Theorists tend to be logical and step-by-step in their approach to learning.

Individuals are most often a combination of the styles – e.g. theorist and reflector, or theorist and pragmatist. If you find out your learning style, it may help you to understand how you learn most effectively both in practice and theory.

In addition to your learning style, Dunn et al. (1989) identify that learning is also influenced by five key factors:

1. Environmental: the learning environment you prefer.
2. Emotional: whether you need motivational support or can learn independently.
3. Sociological: if you work best independently or in a team.
4. Physiological: your preference for visual, auditory or kinaesthetic learning.
5. Psychological: your personal response to information.

ACTIVITY 7.6

Consider each of the five key factors outlined by Dunn et al. (1989) and identify your preferences. Understanding your preferences will help you to analyse how you learn and enable you to develop the most effective approach for you.

There is no definitive answer for this activity as it is personal to the individual.

It is also useful to consider Gardner's 'multiple intelligences' (Gardner, 1983). Gardner proposed that there were seven intelligences and that each individual person has a unique blend. These intelligences are:

- Linguistic intelligence: the ability to learn languages and express yourself.
- Logical-mathematical intelligence: the ability to analyse problems and investigate scientifically.

- Musical intelligence: the ability to perform and appreciate musical patterns.
- Bodily-kinesthetic intelligence: the ability to use the whole body, or parts of it, to solve problems.
- Spatial intelligence: the ability to understand space.
- Interpersonal intelligence: the ability to read other people and communicate with them.
- Intrapersonal intelligence: the ability to understand yourself (self-awareness).

While there is limited evidence in support of multiple intelligences, educationalists, particularly in America, have embraced the concept and used the approach in planning educational programmes. In relation to reflective practice within nursing, it can be helpful to contemplate each of the intelligences.

A further issue to consider, although not strictly a 'learning style', is emotional intelligence (EI). Daniel Goleman (1995) developed the concept of EI, and proposes that it is important in successful leadership. EI comprises five elements:

1. Self-awareness.
2. Self-regulation – e.g. controlling oneself, being self-disciplined.
3. Motivation.
4. Empathy.
5. Social skills – e.g. ability to interact with others.

As nurses, the elements of EI are clearly important, and again there are online tests to identify where on the spectrum you are. Knowing your emotional intelligence enables you to identify strengths and areas for development.

The final theory we will consider in our discussion of concepts related to learning styles is Carper's 'fundamental patterns of knowing' (Carper, 1978). He suggests that there are four areas of knowledge that nurses learn in order to function effectively:

1. Empirical knowing – theoretical knowledge underpinning practice.
2. Aesthetic knowing – the 'art' of nursing, the practical elements surrounding the nursing process, which can be intuitive, recognising the clinical needs for that patient at that time, underpinned by empirical or theoretical knowledge.
3. Personal knowing – e.g. knowing yourself.
4. Ethical knowing – e.g. knowing the morality and ethical elements of nursing.

Johns (2017) developed Carper's ways of knowing into a reflective model. Using this model to reflect will enable you to consider how confident you are in respect of each 'pattern of knowing', thus identifying areas for development.

We have discussed a number of approaches: multiple intelligences by VARK (2019), Honey and Mumford (1992), Dunn et al. (1989) and Gardner (1983); emotional intelligence by Goleman (1995) and ways of knowing by Carper (1978). Insight into your learning style gained through the use of appropriate questionnaires, or consideration of the elements of each style we have identified, can provide insight into learning strengths and developmental needs. Through identifying personal learning styles, it is possible to develop strategies to support your own learning in order to improve practice.

To explain how this can be done we will return to Sam, who we met at the beginning of this chapter, and illustrate how knowing your learning style can support development of practice. To provide some further details about Sam, he is a busy, sports-focused individual, who knows that he is an activist, prefers to learn with others and enjoys learning kinaesthetically. He completed an emotional intelligence test and received a high score, which reassured him that he is empathising and relating effectively to his patients and colleagues. Sam also reviewed Carper's ways of knowing and felt that he is strong in relation to aesthetic, personal and ethical knowledge, but that his empirical knowledge needs developing. In relation to the challenge of reflecting Sam mentioned at the beginning of this chapter, he could use Carper's framework as a model of reflection to consider his strengths and development needs. More generally, Sam could use knowledge of his learning styles to develop his practice by considering that as he tends to be an activist, he frequently maximises every learning opportunity. This is a positive attribute, which is excellent. However, it might also mean that he doesn't always take time to reflect or practise skills, and this is an area where he could develop. Identifying that his empirical knowledge needs to be developed is also helpful, as it will motivate him to find time to study and reduce the gaps in his knowledge. As he knows that he prefers kinaesthetic learning, it will be useful for him to develop his knowledge through observation and practice as much as possible, in addition to reading and writing.

ACTIVITY 7.7

Use an online tool to find out your learning style.

- Consider the results you are given, but remember that you do not have to agree with them, as you may already have a good insight into how you learn best.
- Reflect on the results you were given and, using this plus your knowledge of the way you learn, develop a strategy to maximise your learning in order to develop your practice.

There is no definitive answer for this activity as it is personal to the individual.

CONCLUSION

Self-awareness and knowing oneself honestly as a practitioner are vital for developing practice. Being self-aware in order to improve practice is, however, a complex process. It is important to identify your strengths and limitations through self-analysis, using different 'lenses' as suggested by Brookfield (1998), including feedback from others. It is also helpful to understand your own beliefs and values, as these can impact on your practice, preventing you from remaining objective. Recognition of your learning styles will help you to identify learning strategies for your ongoing development.

GOING FURTHER

Barker, S., Scammell, J., Morgan, G., Santos, A., Johnson, B., Stacey-Emile, G. and Al Battashi, H. (2016) *Psychology for Nursing & Healthcare Professionals. Developing Compassionate Care*. London: Sage. A comprehensive and accessible psychology book for nursing students.

Carper, B. (1978) Fundamental patterns of knowing in nursing. *Advanced Nursing Science*, 1(1): 13-23. A seminal article which is very interesting to read as the ways of knowing underpins so much of our practice.

Howard Gardner's Multiple Intelligences. Go to: www.businessballs.com/howardgardner multipleintelligences.htm#multiple%20intelligences%20tests. A useful site that will help you understand how you learn.

GLOSSARY

acronym   Abbreviation formed from the first letter of each word.

attributes   Qualities or characteristics.

concept   Idea.

context   The circumstances or the situation.

internally driven   Come from within us.

kinaesthetic   Relating to awareness of the position and movement of parts of the body.

notion   Thought.

psychosocial   The interrelation of social factors and individual thought and behaviour.

REFERENCES

Bandura, A. (1977) *Social Learning Theory*. Englewood Cliffs, NJ: Prentice Hall.

Brookfield, S. (1998) Critically reflective practice. *Journal of Continuing Education in the Health Professions*, 18: 197–205.

Brown, G., Leonard, C. and Arthur-Kelly, M. (2016) Writing SMARTER goals for professional learning and improving classroom practices. *Reflective Practice*, 17(5): 621–35.

Carper, B. (1978) Fundamental patterns of knowing in nursing. *Advanced Nursing Science*, 1(1): 13–23.

Dunn, R., Dunn, K. and Price, G.E. (1989) *Learning Style Inventory*. Lawrence, KS: Price Systems.

Gardner, H. (1983) *Frames of Mind: The Theory of Multiple Intelligences*. New York: Basic Books.

Goleman, D. (1995) *Emotional Intelligence*. New York: Bantam Books.

Honey, P. and Mumford, A. (1992) *The Manual of Learning Styles*. Maidenhead: Peter Honey Publications.

Johns, C. (2017) *Becoming a Reflective Practitioner* (5th edn). Chichester: Wiley-Blackwell.

Luft, J. (1969) *Human Interaction*. Palo Alto, CA: National Press.

Moustafa Leonard, K. and Padkil, F. (2016) *Performance Leadership*. New York: Business Expert Press.

NHS (2012) *Compassion in Practice: Nursing, Midwifery and Care Staff Our Vision and Strategy*. Available at: www.england.nhs.uk/wp-content/uploads/2012/12/ compassion-in-practice.pdf (accessed 17 August 2020).

NHS (2015) The NHS Constitution for England. Available at: www.gov.uk/government/ publications/the-nhs-constitution-for-england/the-nhs-constitution-for-england (accessed 20 August 2020).

Oxford Dictionary (2016a) Definition of belief. Available at: https://
en.oxforddictionaries.com/definition/belief (accessed 17 August 2020).

Oxford Dictionary (2016b) Definition of value. Available online at: https://
en.oxforddictionaries.com/definition/value (accessed 17 August 2020).

Paediatric FOAMed (2018) A discussion of the 'Hot Debrief'. Available at: www.
paediatricfoam.com/2017/01/the-hot-debrief/ (accessed 17 August 2020).

Pearce, C. (2007) Ten steps to carrying out a SWOT analysis. *Nursing Management*, 14(2): 25.

VARK (2019) VARK, a guide to learning styles. Available at: http://vark-learn.com
(accessed 17 August 2020).

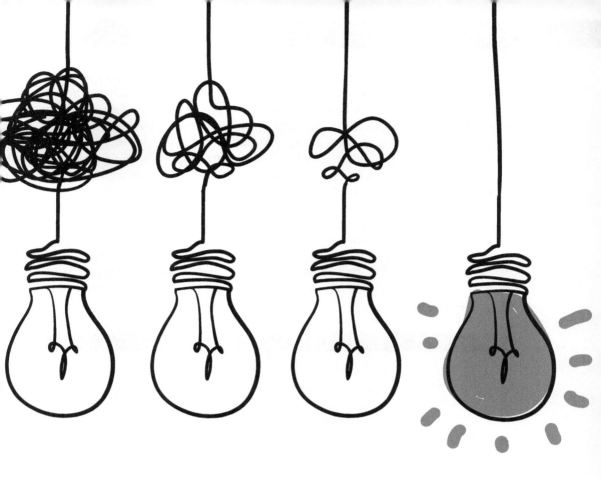

PART C

GOING FURTHER

The final part of the book will enable you to appreciate the wider issues relevant to reflective practice, recognise that experience alone does not result in the ability to deliver the best patient care, consider competency and proficiency, plus introduce you to the concept of nursing intuition. We will highlight the role that reflection has in lifelong learning, plus how reflection links theory and practice. To end this part of the book, we will consider theory and philosophy relevant to reflective practice, identifying the fundamental role that emotion plays in learning, and outlining that there remains further work to be done to fully realise the potential of reflective practice in nursing.

At the start of each chapter you will hear from a registered nurse and nursing student who are very likely to be sharing the challenges and asking the questions you are, as you continue on your journey towards 'being reflective'.

Before you start to read the chapters in this part, however, I would like to introduce you to Rati Patil, who is going to share her thoughts and a reflection with you. As we progress through this part of the book, we will refer back to Rati's work and identify how it could be developed.

CASE STUDY

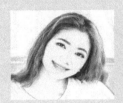

RATI PATIL, THIRD YEAR NURSING STUDENT, LEARNING DISABILITY FIELD

HI! I AM RATI!

I'm a third-year learning disability student and am now on placement on an acute orthopaedic ward within a large regional hospital. I have just started this placement, but in earlier placements I noticed that sometimes patients living with dementia are difficult to communicate with.

Before I started this placement I attended a 'Dementia Friends' session, which has changed how I think about communicating with patients with dementia.

I have focused on this topic in my reflection, considering an experience that was particularly significant for me.

RATI'S REFLECTION

INTRODUCTION

For this reflection, I will use Gibbs's model of reflection (Gibbs, 1988) of description, feelings, evaluation, analysis, conclusion and action plan as I feel it will help me to analyse this critical incident which occurred during the first week of my first placement in my third year.

DESCRIPTION

It was my third shift on the ward, and after the morning handover my mentor and I went to greet all of the patients in our team. One of the patients was 'Mary' - not her real name, anonymised in line with the General Data Protection Regulation (GDPR, 2018). She had just arrived from the Surgical Assessment

Unit (SAU) and we had received a handover from SAU that she was living with dementia and had a fractured neck of femur (NOF), but that was really all. As we entered the bay, we could see that she was confused and distressed about where she was. She kept saying that she needed to get up and go to work. Mary was clearly very frustrated and looked like she might get out of bed, which would not have been ideal due to her fractured NOF. I immediately crouched down next to her so that I was at her eye level and engaged her in a very positive conversation about her work, engaging with her reality sensitively, as this is important for patients living with dementia (Social Care Institute for Excellence, 2015). This helped her to calm down significantly and we talked about the florist shop that she had worked in. Mary settled and after a short while we moved the conversation to what she would like to eat for breakfast. I was then able to leave her to wait for her breakfast, which arrived soon after the end of our conversation.

FEELINGS

I was concerned about Mary's distress and also worried that she might stand up, make her fracture worse and potentially have a fall. I was pleased that I was able to sit down next to her, engage with her and help her to calm down so that she could eat breakfast.

I also felt frustrated and annoyed that we had not received in the handover from SAU that she was confused – their handover was very minimal.

EVALUATION

This incident allowed me to put my communication skills into practice by talking to Mary to reduce her confusion and distress. I consider that I was effective at engaging with Mary's reality and that the conversation supported her emotionally, helping her to feel valued and supported. It also ensured that Mary did not get out of bed. The incident also highlighted that Mary needed a '**special**' to sit with her to ensure that she remained safe.

ANALYSIS

Just before commencing this placement, we had a 'Dementia Friends Information Session' (Alzheimer's Society, 2017). This was interesting and helped me to think more about how I communicate with people living with dementia. One of the key things that stayed in my mind from the Dementia Friends session was that while many people living with dementia may have short-term memory loss related to factual information, their emotional memory might not be affected. In other words, a person with dementia may not remember what was said (the fact), but is likely to remember how it was said (the emotion).

When I was communicating with Mary, I was thinking very much about this emotional element, more than I would have done prior to the Dementia Friends session – e.g. how I wanted Mary to feel valued and listened to, and that I cared. I feel that I communicated with Mary with more compassion and calmness than I might have done on earlier placements, and this enabled Mary to settle down and feel safe.

(Continued)

This experience has also taught me how important it is to assess patients as soon as possible after they arrive, even if you have a handover. It is important to assess for yourself, and read medical notes in case anything has been missed, or the patient has perhaps deteriorated since the handover.

CONCLUSION

This experience has shown how important it is to take time to speak to people living with dementia and to speak to them in a supportive way so they feel valued. This, of course, is true for all patients, but for patients living with dementia, it seems even more important, as while they may not remember what you have said, they are likely to remember how you made them feel.

It also highlighted the importance of early and ongoing patient assessment, and reading a patient's notes, to ensure that you have as full a picture of the person as possible, as soon as they come into your care.

ACTION PLAN

It was good to attend the 'Dementia Friends' information session, as it helped me to communicate with Mary. In future, I will think about how I make a person feel when I talk to them, whether they are living with dementia or not.

The experience has also highlighted how interested I am in communicating with people with dementia and how I have observed that sometimes it can be improved. I am going to focus on this area for my dissertation as I would like to understand how we can improve communication within the acute setting for patients living with dementia.

I will also ensure that I always assess my patients as soon as they are under my care.

GLOSSARY

special   When a patient's condition needs one member of the healthcare team to remain with them at all times.

REFERENCES

Alzheimer's Society (2017) Dementia Friends. Available at: www.dementiafriends.org.uk/ (accessed 18 August 2020).

General Data Protection Regulation (2018). Data Protection Act 2018, c. 12. Available at: www.legislation.gov.uk/ukpga/2018/12/contents/enacted (accessed 27 October 2020).

Gibbs, G. (1988) *Learning by Doing: A Guide to Teaching and Learning Methods.* Further Education Unit, Oxford Polytechnic, Oxford.

Social Care Institute for Excellence (2015) Dementia: When people with dementia experience a different reality. Available at: www.scie.org.uk/dementia/living-with-dementia/difficult-situations/different-reality.asp (accessed 18 August 2020).

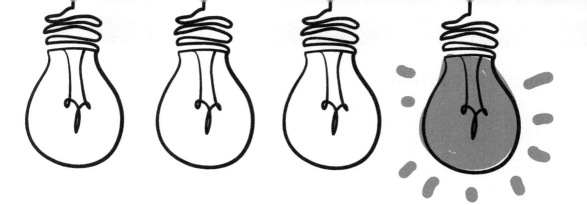

ACHIEVING AND MAINTAINING COMPETENCE THROUGH REFLECTION

CORAL DRANE

> " I am nearly qualified – how scary! For my final portfolio I have to include a reflection related to the NMC *Code* and proficiencies. How am I going to do that?
>
> **Hannah Bride, nursing student, adult field** "

> " I have to revalidate soon. I know that there are reflection forms to complete as I have been to a revalidation study day, but I am still worried. I would like to reflect on my competence in managing the ward, now that I am 'in charge', but this sounds very broad? Would this be possible?
>
> **Colin Grace, registered nurse, adult field** "

INTRODUCTION

As nurses and nursing students, we constantly have to ensure that we are working in line with the NMC (2018c) *Code* and are proficient and competent in our practice. Revalidation is integral to this and, as Colin says at the beginning of this chapter, writing about competence within our role is a good area for reflection, and as Hannah identifies, nursing students are often asked to reflect on proficiencies for an assessment.

Reflecting on competency and proficiency are important elements for reflection. In this chapter we will examine competence and proficiency, and how reflecting on these can assist the achievement of competence as a nursing student and its maintenance as a registered nurse.

First, we will explore what is meant by competence and proficiency, from the perspective of both a nursing student and a registered nurse. Theories and professional codes relating to competence will be considered and methods of measuring competence will be discussed. Reflection to demonstrate competency for revalidation will then be highlighted, and the integral role that reflection plays in lifelong learning will conclude the chapter. Throughout the chapter we will draw on the experiences of Rati Patil, who we met in Part C, as well as Hannah and Colin, who we heard from at the start of the chapter.

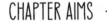 CHAPTER AIMS

This chapter will enable to you to:

- understand what we mean by 'competency' and 'proficiency' and how these can be measured;
- explore theoretical models and frameworks of 'competency' and 'proficiency';
- appreciate the role of reflection in becoming competent;
- realise how reflection can be used to demonstrate competence for revalidation;
- recognise the overarching role of reflection in lifelong learning.

WHAT DO WE MEAN BY COMPETENCY AND PROFICIENCY IN NURSING?

There are many definitions for competency and proficiency, but maybe the simplest is that competency is 'the ability to do something well' and 'a skill that you need in a particular job or for a particular task' and proficiency is 'the ability to do something well because of training and practice' (Oxford University Press, 2020).

How these definitions relate to nursing, whether proficiency is a progression of competency, or if competency and proficiency can be considered parallel in terms of ability, however, remains unclear.

Benner (1984) developed a framework for clinical competency which proposed that 'competency' proceeds 'proficiency'. Benner's framework, based on Dreyfus and Dreyfus (1980) is summarised in Table 8.1 and suggests that as nurses develop their skill, they progress through the five stages.

Table 8.1   From novice to expert

Stage	Name	Performance
1.	Novice	Has no experience and lacks confidence in the situation they are in. Needs to be coached continuously and is not able to make any judgements.
2.	Advanced beginner	Acceptable performance based on previous experiences but still needs occasional coaching and support. Is skilful in some areas and has developing knowledge.
3.	Competent	Is confident in their actions, and is efficient and co-ordinated in their work. No longer needs any support.
4.	Proficient	Is holistic in their approach, rather than viewing situations in parts. Has learned from experience and is able to plan and respond to events appropriately and in a timely manner.
5.	Expert	Has an intuitive grasp and a deep understanding of situations. Is able to act very quickly with a high level of proficiency even in situations that they have not experienced before.

Source: Benner (1984) From novice to expert, excellence and power in clinical nursing practice, pp. 13-34. Adapted with kind permission of John Wiley & Sons.

Benner's stages of development may be simplistic, and it is possible to be an 'advanced beginner' in some processes and 'expert' in others. Nonetheless, these stages are well recognised and provide a valuable **conceptual framework** for nursing skill **acquisition**.

ACTIVITY 8.1

Consider Benner's stages of development.

- Where would you place yourself in respect of your nursing skills?
- Are you are at the same point with all your skills or are you at different stages in different skills?

Check the activity answers at the end of the chapter to see if our thoughts are similar.

The terms 'competency' and 'proficiency' have both been used in relation to Nursing and Midwifery Council (NMC) standards for nursing. Historically, the term 'competency' was used, but 'proficiency' standards for registered nurses have now been published to reflect the role of the nurse in the twenty-first century (NMC, 2018a). These replace the NMC competency standards that were published in 2014. The publication of competency standards in 2014 was to satisfy demands by the public for more transparency and information relating to nursing standards. This came in the aftermath of the Francis Report (Crown Copyright, 2013a), and the *More Care, Less Pathway* report into the workings of the Liverpool Care Pathway (Crown Copyright, 2013b).

The 2018 NMC proficiency standards (NMC, 2018a) is a framework for pre-registration nursing education, and standards for student supervision and assessment (NMC, 2018b). It is interesting that the NMC has replaced the term 'competency' with 'proficiency' in their current standards and raises the question as to whether there is an expectation for nurses to be more skilled on qualification. Indeed, a greater number of enhanced clinical skills are required within the 2018 NMC proficiencies. This change in terminology may also reflect the cultural shift towards transparency and openness in the wake of the Francis Report (Crown Copyright, 2013a) and also the drive to improve standards championed via the Care Quality Commission (CQC).

Alongside the competency and proficiency standards, nurses are required to abide by *The Code* (NMC, 2018c) throughout their career. Failure to meet the standards or to abide by *The Code* results in not only poor patient care, but also an NMC investigation into a registered nurse's fitness to practise, and could mean that a person is removed from the nursing register. Thus, maintaining competency is fundamentally important.

Nursing students are constantly working towards competency and proficiency throughout their nursing programme and are assessed against **learning outcomes** linked directly to the NMC standards and code. Thus, competency and proficiency are fundamentally important for nursing students, too.

The 2018 NMC standards of proficiency for nurses are more complex than previous versions and have seven 'platforms' that apply to all registered nurses. In addition to the seven platforms are two annexes, which contain proficiencies for all registered nurses. These annexes are: A) communication and relationship management skills, and B) nursing procedures. Table 8.2 illustrates the seven platforms (NMC, 2018a).

Table 8.2   Seven platforms, Standards of proficiency

Platform 1	Being an accountable professional.
Platform 2	Promoting health and preventing ill health.
Platform 3	Assessing needs and planning care.
Platform 4	Providing and evaluating care.
Platform 5	Leading and managing nursing care and working in teams.
Platform 6	Improving safety and quality of care.
Platform 7	Coordinating care.

Source: Adapted from NMC (2018a)

These 2018 Standards (NMC, 2018a, pp. 9, 13 and 21) make a number of references to reflection – in Platform 1 as part of the overarching outcome statement: 'Registered nurses continually reflect on their practice and keep abreast of new and emerging developments in nursing, health and care.'

Within Platforms 1, 5 and 6, and Annexe A they state:

1.14   provide and promote non-discriminatory, person-centred and sensitive care at all times, *reflecting* on people's values and beliefs, diverse backgrounds, cultural characteristics, language requirements, needs and preferences, taking account of any need for adjustments

1.17   take responsibility for continuous *self-reflection*, seeking and responding to support and feedback to develop their professional knowledge and skills

5.8   support and supervise students in the delivery of nursing care, *promoting reflection* and providing constructive feedback, and evaluating and documenting their performance

5.10   contribute to supervision and *team reflection* activities to promote improvements in practice and services

6.8   demonstrate an understanding of how to identify, report and *critically reflect* on near misses, critical incidents, major incidents and serious adverse events in order to learn from them and influence their future practice

From Annexe A: Communication and relationship management skills:

4.1.4   demonstrate effective supervision, teaching and performance appraisal through the use of: encouragement to colleagues that helps them to *reflect* on their practice

Thus, reflection is clearly considered by the NMC to be important in supporting competency and proficiency.

ACTIVITY 8.2

Consider the seven proficiency platforms in Table 8.2.

- Could you use these platforms as a way to focus a reflection and identify your level of competence?
- Would this be a useful process?

Check the activity answers at the end of the chapter to see if our thoughts on this are similar.

THEORIES AND FRAMEWORKS OF COMPETENCY AND PROFICIENCY

As we have discussed, the proficiencies identified by the NMC need to be achieved within nursing pre-registration education, and maintained and developed following registration. Benner (1984) provides us with a valuable framework showing how skill is developed and is a potential tool for reflection, but other competency models are also worthy of consideration.

One of the most commonly quoted competency models is the conscious competence learning model (Broadwell, 1969). This model proposes that individuals progress through four stages in learning:

1. *Unconscious incompetence:* a person doesn't know what they don't know – e.g. they are not conscious of the skill that they need to learn. In the nursing context, a beginning student who has never been a health care assistant, is likely to be unaware of the skills that they will need to learn when starting their first placement.
2. *Conscious incompetence:* a person realises that they need to learn something new – e.g. a nursing student is asked to catheterise a patient but doesn't know how, so they are conscious of their incompetence.
3. *Conscious competence:* a person has now consciously learned something and is competent at it, but has to focus and think about how to do it – e.g. a nursing student has learned how to insert a catheter and is competent at this skill, but has to think about how to do it to be successful.
4. *Unconscious competence:* a person can now do the skill they have learned without having to think about it and it has become automatic. In the term used by Benner (1984), they have become an expert – e.g. a registered nurse has inserted numerous catheters during their practice and the process is automatic for them.

There is potentially a fifth level in this model (Businessballs, 2020). This could be:

5. *Reflective competence:* a person is able to 'unpick' their achievement of level 4, unconscious competence. What this means is, for example, that an experienced nurse would be able to 'deconstruct' how they insert a catheter, as they have expert understanding of every aspect of the process. They could reflect on how effective they had been each time they catheterised and be able to teach the skill to others. Achieving 'reflective competence' ensures that competence is maintained, and indeed improved, and also enables the mentoring of a colleague.

A further model that can be used to measure competence is Bloom's taxonomy (Bloom et al., 1956). It is shown in Figure 8.1 and, essentially, provides a hierarchical framework of developing competence in all three learning domains applicable to nursing: psychomotor (skills), cognitive (knowledge) and affective (attitude).

Bloom's Domains of Learning
(higher order skills are on top)

Psychomotor	Cognitive	Affective
• Origination	• Evaluation	• Characterizing
• Adaptation	• Synthesis	• Organizing
• Complex Overt Response	• Analysis	• Valuing
• Mechanism	• Application	• Responding
• Guided Response	• Comprehension	• Receiving
• Set	• Knowledge	
• Perception		

Figure 8.1   Bloom's taxonomy

Source: Bloom's taxonomy (1956). Images from NICHE (2018), created by Esther Isabelle Wilder. Reproduced with kind permission of Esther Isabelle Wilder.

It is useful to consider Bloom's taxonomy as it refers to competency not only in skills, but also in knowledge and attitude. The consideration of all three of these areas makes it particularly valuable, as nurses need not only to be competent in how they undertake skills, but they also need a sound knowledge base to support their skills and an appropriate attitude.

ACTIVITY 8.3

Consider the competency models identified in this chapter.

- Which model do you find most useful?
- Can you relate Bloom's three domains to your development?

There is no definitive answer to this activity as the questions are based on your own perspective.

THE ROLE OF REFLECTION IN BECOMING COMPETENT

Achieving and maintaining competence and proficiency against the NMC Standards and *Code* is vital in nursing, and reflection should be used to support this.

In Chapter 1, reflection was discussed as a way of learning through experience or thinking with a purpose. In the context of becoming competent and maintaining competency, reflection can be used to help assess whether the required competencies and proficiencies are being achieved. At the start of the chapter, Hannah told us that she has to produce a reflection related to the NMC *Code* and proficiencies. As you will see from 'Hannah's reflection', she chose to reflect on an experience relating to the specific proficiency 1.14 from the NMC Standards (2018a, p. 6):

1.14   provide and promote non-discriminatory, person-centred and sensitive care at all times, *reflecting* on people's values and beliefs, diverse backgrounds, cultural characteristics, language requirements, needs and preferences, taking account of any need for adjustments

This proficiency also clearly links to the first element of the NMC *Code*, 'Prioritise people' (NMC, 2018c).

CASE STUDY 8.1

HANNAH'S REFLECTION

Title: Reflection related to the first element of the NMC (2018a) *Code* 'Prioritise people' and the NMC (2018b) Standard (proficiency 1.14):

(Continued)

provide and promote non-discriminatory, person-centred and sensitive care at all times, reflecting on people's values and beliefs, diverse backgrounds, cultural characteristics, language requirements, needs and preferences, taking account of any need for adjustments

In this reflection, I will use Borton's simple reflective model of 'What?, So what?, Now what?' (Borton, 1970), but I will also refer to the competency framework proposed originally by Broadwell (1969) (terms in italics), which suggests that we progress through the following stages: *unconscious incompetence, conscious incompetence, conscious competence and unconscious competence.*

WHAT?

During my final placement, I looked after a patient 'John' (not his real name, pseudonym used to preserve confidentiality, NMC, 2018a). John was a prisoner from the local prison. He was friendly and approachable, and I found him easy to relate to and care for. It was hard to imagine that he was a prisoner and has done something serious enough to be sent to prison.

SO WHAT?

I have learned about my prejudices and assumptions through looking after John. Prior to looking after him I was *unconsciously incompetent* with regard to caring for a prisoner. I had not met a prisoner before and hadn't really thought about this. If I had thought about it, I would have assumed that I would find it difficult to look after them, that I might feel angry towards them, or discriminate against them unwittingly because of their prisoner status, even though I know I should be non-judgemental (NMC, 2018a).

When I first started looking after John, I was *consciously incompetent* as I was very nervous about how I would approach him. I felt clumsy in my communication with him and was unsure about my feelings towards him. However, very quickly as I developed a therapeutic relationship with him, I became *consciously competent* in my communication and care for John. I realised that I wasn't prejudiced at all; in fact, I was able to develop a good rapport with him, and didn't think about his background or discriminate in any way against him.

NOW WHAT?

I feel that my care for John was non-discriminatory and person-centred (NMC, 2018b). I did not need to challenge anyone else's discrimination against John, but would have felt able to do so if needed.

When I next look after a prisoner, I will be *consciously competent* in the process, even if the prisoner is not as approachable as John. I will not feel as nervous to approach them, and know that the fact that they are a prisoner will not impact on my care or behaviour towards them.

REFERENCES

Borton, T. (1970) *Reach, Touch and Teach*. London: Hutchinson.

Broadwell, M.M. (1969) Teaching for learning (XVI). *Gospel Guardian*, 20(41): 1–3a.

NMC (2018a) *The Code*. London: NMC.

NMC (2018b) Standards of proficiency for registered nurses. Available at: www.nmc.
org.uk/standards/standards-for-nurses/standards-of-proficiency-for-registered-nurses/
(accessed 18 August 2020).

ACTIVITY 8.4

Read Hannah's reflection.

- Was it useful to use the competency framework proposed originally by Broadwell (1969) or would another framework have been better?
- Could Hannah have related her reflection to any other NMC (2018a) standards or to any other elements of the NMC (2018c) *Code*?

Check the activity answers at the end of the chapter to see if our thoughts are similar.

To consider further how we can use reflection as a way to demonstrate competency, if we review the reflection written by Rati Patil in Part C, as Rati is talking to us, she is subconsciously reflecting on her growing competency and proficiency relating to communication, specifically surrounding her communication with patients living with dementia. The NMC proficiencies (2018a, pp. 27–30) highlight the importance of communication within Annexe A, and it is clear that in her reflection Rati is conscious of her competence in relation to using a person-centred approach to communication. Rati also identifies how she plans to develop learning related to communication by focusing her dissertation on improving communication for people living with dementia in the acute setting. In her reflection, even though Rati has not explicitly discussed competency or proficiency, she is reflecting implicitly upon her development towards communication proficiency.

Rati and Hannah have shown how it is possible to reflect both explicitly and implicitly on NMC proficiencies. Reflections like these are a very common way of assessing how pre-registration nursing students relate theory to practice as they become proficient.

Levett-Jones (2007) identified that frequently when nursing students write, what they produce is interspersed with competencies. As we have seen, this was true in Rati's case.

Using this approach, outlined in more detail in Figure 8.2, provides an excellent way to self-assess competencies.

Although this process is very detailed, it provides a useful tool specifically for self-assessment against competencies and proficiencies that need to be achieved and maintained in nursing.

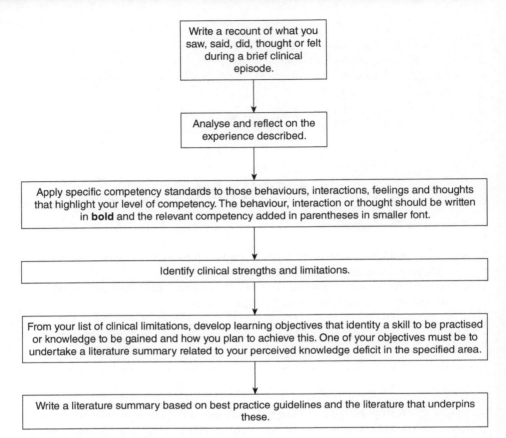

Figure 8.2   Flowchart of the nursing narrative

Source: Levett-Jones, T. (2007) Facilitating reflective practice and self-assessment of competence through the use of narratives. *Nurse Education in Practice*, 7: 112–19. Reproduced with kind permission of Elsevier.

ACTIVITY 8.5

Review Figure 8.2 above.

- Find a reflection you have written recently and apply this process to it.
- Did it help you to identify any developments against a specific competency or proficiency?

There is no definitive answer for this activity as it is personal to you, but you could discuss what you have written with a colleague, your practice supervisor or university lecturer.

As we have said, reflection is frequently used as a way to assess nursing students' competence and ability to achieve learning outcomes. This is an important aspect of achieving and maintaining competency, and it must be ensured that the new knowledge gained from the process is applied to practice.

THE ROLE OF REFLECTION IN REVALIDATION

Revalidation is how registered nurses provide evidence every three years that they are maintaining their competence. This is done by recording their continuous professional development (CPD), obtaining practice-related feedback, and through writing five reflections linked to the CPD they have undertaken, practice-related feedback, or any other event or experience (NMC, 2019). As part of revalidation there is also a reflective discussion with an NMC registered colleague (NMC, 2019).

We met Colin at the beginning of this chapter and he was worrying out his imminent revalidation, and wondering if he could write a reflection on his competence to manage the ward as nurse in charge. Figure 8.3 shows the reflection that he wrote, using the NMC (2019) format.

REFLECTIVE ACCOUNTS FORM

You must use this form to record five written reflective accounts on your CPD and/or practice-related feedback and/or an event or experience in your practice and how this relates to the Code. Please fill in a page for each of your reflective accounts, making sure you do not include any information that might identify a specific patient, service user, colleague or other individuals. Please refer to our guidance on preserving anonymity in the section on non-identifiable information in *How to revalidate with the NMC*.

Reflective account:
What was the nature of the CPD activity and/or practice-related feedback and/or event or experience in your practice?
This reflection will be about my competence to manage the ward on a typical day when I am 'Nurse in Charge (NIC)'. The day that I am going to reflect on was a Saturday, when I was NIC of our general medical ward and had to co-ordinate beds as well as support colleagues within the 37 bedded ward. I will reflect applying Benner's (1984) competency framework in relation to the different aspects of my ward management.
The day was an average day, where I had to communicate continually via telephone, with the Site Team about the bed status, and update them with discharges as there was a lot of pressure on the hospital 'front door' in A & E. To remain up to date myself on the bed status, I had to check in with four staff nurses on the ward in charge of each team of 9 or 10 patients to find out how near to discharge they were with each patient due for discharge, and also support them with extra clinical elements, such as cannulation, phlebotomy, blood transfusions, IVs, etc.
It is always a continual 'juggle' of communication in all directions.

(Continued)

Figure 8.3 (Continued)

What did you learn from the CPD activity and/or feedback and/or event or experience in your practice?

This was a fairly average Saturday with 7 patients to discharge on the ward, two relatively newly qualified nurses on shift, and two experienced staff nurses. I learned on this day that although I feel I am quite an inexperienced NIC, within the medical ward setting (I have changed from being a surgical nurse to a medical nurse recently) I coped well with the 'juggling' of communication between colleagues. Relating to Benner's (1984) stages of development I feel that I was 'proficient' in terms of the communication elements of the day, which helps me feel positive my ability to function in the NIC role.

In relation to my ability to carry out clinical skills to support my colleagues, I found this more difficult, due to the demands of constant phone calls. It was difficult to prioritise these clinical skills in a timely way, as I was being phoned so often. In respect of Benner's (1984) stages, I was an advanced beginner, possibly verging on the competent with the support element of the role.

How did you change or improve your practice as a result?

Through this reflection I can see that I need to improve my competence relating to how I support my colleagues when I am NIC. I could do this by being more assertive with the phone calls to allow me to carve out more time to support colleagues, particularly those who are quite newly qualified. I could potentially support the newly qualified nurses specifically by helping them to learn to delegate more, so they have more space themselves to manage. I will also talk to more experienced colleagues and ask them for advice about how they are able to successfully fulfil both parts of the NIC role.

How is this relevant to the Code?

Select one or more themes: Prioritise people – Practise effectively – Preserve safety – Promote professionalism and trust

This reflection links to the code primarily in relation to 'Practise effectively'; e.g. 7. Communicate clearly, 8. Work co-operatively, 9. Share your skills, knowledge and experience for the benefit of people receiving care and your colleagues, and 11. Be accountable for your decisions to delegate tasks and duties to other people. It also relates to leadership within 'Promote professionalism and trust': 25. Provide leadership to make sure people's wellbeing is protected and to improve their experiences of the health and care system.

Figure 8.3 Colin's reflective accounts form

It is clear from this reflection that Colin has considered his competency in relation to his role as nurse in charge and identified supporting colleagues as an area for development. As part of the revalidation process, as well as reflecting on an experience, it is possible to choose an area of *The Code* that you feel you would like to develop and reflect in relation to it. In Colin's case, perhaps he could specifically reflect in relation to the NMC *Code* (2018c):

> 9.4   support students' and colleagues' learning to help them develop their professional competence and confidence.

There are endless possibilities for revalidation reflections, and it is a very positive opportunity for individuals to value their achievements, self-assess and maintain competencies.

REFLECTION AS A VALUABLE LEARNING TOOL

Reflection has the potential to assist in the identification of learning needs through the constant 'unpicking' of situations. Edwards (2014, p. 2) suggests that story-telling can be used alongside reflection to identify **tacit knowledge** – e.g. knowledge unconsciously gained in the workplace, which is difficult to identify. She suggests that through the telling of a story to colleagues, alongside reflection, gaps in knowledge may be more effectively identified.

If we consider this in respect of the reflective discussion that is part of the NMC revalidation process, this may allow an opportunity for story-telling to identify further learning needs not already identified through the five reflective accounts.

ACTIVITY 8.6

Consider the idea of 'story-telling' as a way of adding to your reflection.

- Would you find story-telling a valuable contribution to your reflective processes?
- Would a verbal or written story be preferable for you?

Check the activity answers at the end of the chapter to see if our thoughts are similar.

THE OVERARCHING ROLE OF REFLECTION IN LIFELONG LEARNING

Lifelong learning is a term that has been used consistently over the past 30 years and has many definitions. Longworth and Davis (2003, p. 22) provide a useful summary of lifelong learning as the

> *development of human potential through a continuously supportive process which stimulates and empowers individuals to acquire all the knowledge, values, skills, and understanding they will require throughout their lifetimes and to apply them with confidence, creativity and enjoyment in all roles, circumstances and environments.*

In a study, Davis et al. (2014) identified that lifelong learning was a dynamic process involving personal and professional roles, through both formal and informal learning, with the essential characteristics for successful lifelong learning being reflection, questioning, enjoying learning, understanding of the dynamic nature of knowledge and engaging in learning by seeking learning opportunities. In the study, reflection was ranked as the most important characteristic for effective lifelong learning.

CONCLUSION

When we consider competency and proficiency, upholding the NMC (2018c) *Code*, and achieving and maintaining the NMC (2018a) standards must remain at the forefront of our minds.

Reflection can be used to demonstrate competency and proficiency against competencies, and also as a tool for learning and development. It is also a fundamentally important aspect in lifelong learning.

GOING FURTHER

Bolton, G. with Delderfield, R. (2018) *Reflective Practice, Writing and Professional Development* (5th edn). London: Sage. An excellent book with many useful chapters, including a very informative chapter about 'The Power of the Narrative' which links to the use of stories in reflection.

Edwards, S. (2017) Reflecting differently. New dimensions: reflection-before-action and reflection-beyond-action. *International Practice Development Journal*, 7(1): 1–14. This article explores the four stages of reflection as discussed in this chapter.

Conscious competence. Go to: www.balls.com/self-awareness/conscious-competence-learning-model/. This link considers the conscious competence model in detail.

ANSWERS TO ACTIVITIES

Activity 8.1

- As this is individual to you, it is not possible to comment.
- You will undoubtedly find that you will be at different stages of development for different elements of your practice, and this is completely normal. If you are a nursing student, you could consider using Benner's framework for successive placements and develop a map of your development in each area of your practice.

Activity 8.2

- It is possible to do this, and it would help you to identify your areas of strengths, and limitations (as explored in Chapter 7) and then develop an action plan prior to each placement.
- It would be very useful, and undertaking this exercise would also consolidate your understanding of the proficiency platforms that underpin professional practice.

Activity 8.4

- The competency framework proposed originally by Broadwell (1969) was effective within Hannah's reflection, but she could equally have used Benner's framework, although it would have changed the reflection significantly. There are many other frameworks she could have used – the affective domain of Bloom, for example.
- There are so many standards and elements of the *Code*, and so many others also relate to this experience – for example, other outcomes in Platform 1, Being an accountable professional:

  1.11 communicate effectively using a range of skills and strategies with colleagues and people at all stages of life and with a range of mental, physical, cognitive and behavioural health challenges

1.12 demonstrate the skills and abilities required to support people at all stages of life who are emotionally or physically vulnerable

1.13 demonstrate the skills and abilities required to develop, manage and maintain appropriate relationships with people, their families, carers and colleagues.

Hannah has also covered elements of the NMC *Code*, specifically item 7, Communicate clearly, which is within the section 'Practise effectively'.

Activity 8.6

- You might find that you 'story-tell' naturally when talking about your experiences to colleagues. When you find this happening, try to hold on to the ideas and use them in connection with your reflections.
- Verbal story-telling can be a very valuable way to talk through worries and concerns; it can also help you to 'unpick' situations. Writing down the stories will mean that you are more likely to remember and learn from the experiences in the future.

GLOSSARY

acquisition   The learning and development of a skill.

conceptual framework   Organises ideas about a specific topic demonstrating how they relate to each other.

learning outcomes   What a learner will know and be able to do at the end of their programme.

tacit knowledge   Personal knowledge obtained as a result of the direct interaction between individuals and their environment – most people don't recognise their own tacit knowledge.

REFERENCES

Benner, P. (1984) *From Novice to Expert: Excellence and Power in Clinical Nursing Practice*. Menlo Park, CA: Addison-Wesley.

Bloom, B.S., Engelhart, M.D., Furst, E.J., Hill, W.H. and Krathwohl, D.R. (1956) *Taxonomy of Educational Objectives: The Classification of Educational Goals. Handbook I: Cognitive Domain*. New York: David McKay Company.

Broadwell, M.M. (1969) Teaching for learning (XVI). *Gospel Guardian*, 20(41): 1–3a.

Businessballs (2020) Conscious competence learning model. Available at: www.businessballs.com/self-awareness/conscious-competence-learning-model/ (accessed 18 August 2020).

Crown copyright (2013a) The Mid Staffordshire NHS Foundation Trust Public Inquiry Chaired by Robert Francis QC HC 947 Report of the Mid Staffordshire NHS Foundation Trust Public Inquiry Executive summary. Available at: https://assets.publishing.service.gov.uk/government/uploads/system/uploads/attachment_data/file/279124/0947.pdf (accessed 18 August 2020).

Crown copyright (2013b) More Care, Less Pathway report into the workings of the Liverpool Care Pathway. Available at: https://assets.publishing.service.gov.uk/

government/uploads/system/uploads/attachment_data/file/212450/Liverpool_Care_
Pathway.pdf (accessed 18 August 2020).

Davis, L., Taylor, H. and Reyes, H. (2014) Lifelong learning in nursing: A Delphi study. *Nurse Education Today*, pp. 441–5.

Dreyfus, H.L. and Dreyfus, S.E. (1980) A Five-Stage Model of the Mental Activities involved in Directed Skill Acquisition. Available at: www.dtic.mil/dtic/tr/fulltext/u2/a084551.pdf (accessed 18 August 2020).

Edwards, S. (2014) Finding a place for story: looking beyond reflective practice. *International Practice Development Journal*, 4(2): 1–14.

Levett-Jones, T. (2007) Facilitating reflective practice and self-assessment of competence through the use of narratives. *Nurse Education in Practice*, 7: 112–19.

Longworth, N. and Davies, W.K. (2003) *Lifelong Learning* (2nd edn). In Guthrie, J. (ed.), *Encyclopaedia of Education*, Vol. 4. Cleveland, OH: Thomson Gale.

Oxford University Press (2020) Definition of competence. Available at: www.oxfordlearnersdictionaries.com/definition/english/competency?q=competency (accessed 18 August 2020).

Oxford University Press (2020) Definition of proficiency. Available at: www.oxfordlearnersdictionaries.com/definition/english/proficiency?q=proficiency (accessed 18 August 2020).

NICHE (2018) Quantitative reasoning learning goals. Available at: https://serc.carleton.edu/NICHE/qr_learning_goals.html (accessed 18 August 2020).

Nursing and Midwifery Council (NMC) (2018a) Standards of proficiency for registered nurses. Available at: www.nmc.org.uk/standards/standards-for-nurses/standards-of-proficiency-for-registered-nurses/ (accessed 18 August 2020).

NMC (2018b) Part 2: Standards for student supervision and assessment. Available at: www.nmc.org.uk/standards-for-education-and-training/standards-for-student-supervision-and-assessment/ (accessed 18 August 2020).

NMC (2018c) *The Code*. London: NMC.

NMC (2019) Revalidation/resources: Forms and templates. Available at: http://revalidation.nmc.org.uk/download-resources/forms-and-templates/index.html (accessed 18 August 2020).

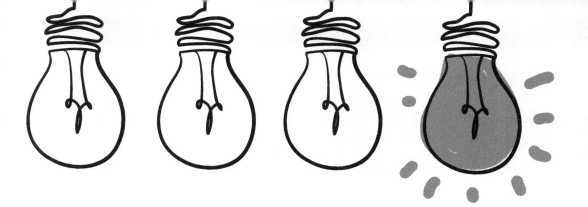

THE ROLE OF REFLECTION IN EVIDENCE-BASED PRACTICE

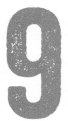

CATHERINE DELVES-YATES

> " I'm confused! In a lecture it was said that reflection is important in evidence-based practice. I can understand the importance of applying the science-based approach of evidence-based practice when treating patients, but where does reflection fit in to this?
>
> **Jean Hunt, nursing student, adult field** "

> " I had an experience last week, when I 'just knew' that one of my patients was becoming increasingly unwell, even though none of their assessments identified this . . . and I was proved right, their condition did deteriorate.
>
> What I can't explain is how I 'just knew' this.
>
> **Samantha Tiler, registered nurse, mental health field** "

INTRODUCTION

Jean is absolutely right. In her comment at the start of the chapter she outlines that evidence-based practice is important in nursing. It most certainly is. Evidence-based practice is the way that we deliver accountable, professional nursing care. As Jean outlines, there is an important scientific or research-based aspect in this, but reflection also has an integral role in ensuring that we apply this knowledge in the most effective way.

Reflection is important in understanding evidence, developing new (research) evidence and strengthening the link between nursing theory and nursing practice. Also, as we will see when we consider what Samantha describes, by reflecting on experience we develop our own personal evidence for nursing. This can assist us to predict changes in a patient's condition.

In this chapter we are going to consider the role that reflection plays in both evidence and evidence-based practice. We will discuss how reflection is fundamental in developing nursing expertise and linking theory with practice, plus consider how reflecting on an experience can lead to undertaking a research project.

--------------------------------- CHAPTER AIMS ---------------------------------

This chapter will enable you to:

- understand the role that reflection plays in evidence-based practice and how it ensures effective care;
- comprehend the importance of developing and applying nursing expertise to patient care;
- recognise that experience alone does not result in the ability to deliver the best patient care;
- define nursing intuition;
- appreciate how reflection on practice can result in research questions;
- realise the role that reflection plays in linking theory and practice.

REFLECTION AS EVIDENCE AND REFLECTION ON EVIDENCE-BASED PRACTICE

As we have discussed in previous chapters, reflection fosters a 'spirit of enquiry' in practitioners, challenging us to examine our actions, enabling us to see how we act and to learn from this new insight. Thus, the experience we gain from caring for patients is important, but reflecting on this is of greater importance. Experience alone does not necessarily lead to learning; it is reflection that makes sense of experience. Reflection makes an experience meaningful and **facilitates** the development of 'personal evidence'. Applying a reflective approach to practice enables us to develop both our individual nursing expertise and our clinical judgement, ensuring that we have some of the tools required to provide the best possible care for patients.

In order to deliver the best possible care, however, there is the need to use further tools, not just reflection alone. We need the ability to base our nursing actions on the most up-to-date scientific (research) evidence available. We also need to be able to adapt our nursing actions to accommodate a patient's experiences, values and expectations.

What we are actually considering here – the scientific evidence, our nursing expertise and the patient perspective – are the three elements which, when combined, create evidence-based practice.

ACTIVITY 9.1

Before reading any further, make a note of how you would explain evidence-based practice to a non-nursing friend.

Check the activity answers at the end of the chapter to see if our thoughts are similar.

EVIDENCE AND EVIDENCE-BASED PRACTICE

To understand evidence-based practice, we need first to consider what we mean by evidence. Evidence can be defined as the knowledge and information we use to help us to make effective decisions. Evidence can come in a range of different forms, but essentially it is the facts or information that indicates whether a belief or proposal is true or valid. In both everyday life and in nursing practice, in order to make any decision, you apply a wide range of information and facts (evidence) from differing sources. You do this by considering the relevant literature, your personal observations (reflections) and the experiences, values and expectations of others (Thorpe and Delves-Yates, 2018).

Relating this more explicitly to nursing, it is when the three elements of

1. external evidence (facts and information from the relevant literature, frequently derived from research and scientific studies),
2. your nursing expertise (which includes your learning from reflection), and
3. the patient's experiences, values and expectations

are combined that we consider ourselves to be applying evidence-based practice. This is shown in Figure 9.1. Evidence-based practice is the way that we deliver accountable, professional nursing care.

Referring to Jean's question at the start of the chapter, she asked what role reflection plays in the science-based approach of evidence-based practice; the answer has to be a fundamental one. Our nursing expertise is based on the experience we gain from caring for patients, but it is reflection on this experience that is the key. Experience on its own does not necessarily lead to learning. It is possible to have many years of nursing experience but still deliver poor patient care. Only by reflecting on the experiences gained during these years, making sense of what happened, learning from this and applying the resulting knowledge to nursing actions, can experience be turned into the ability to deliver excellent patient care.

Thus, reflection is an integral aspect of the **triad of evidence-base practice**, because our nursing expertise comprises the knowledge and experience we have gained from caring for patients previously and, most importantly, learning by reflecting on these experiences. This is what comprises our personal evidence, which is an important form of nursing knowledge.

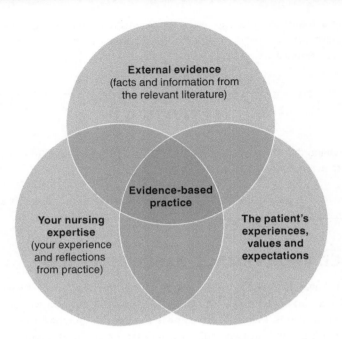

Figure 9.1 Evidence-based practice: the combination of external evidence, nursing expertise and the patient's experiences, values and expectations

Considering further the role that reflection plays with regard to evidence-based practice, if you review Figure 9.1 you will notice that each of the three elements of evidence-based practice are presented in the same-sized shape, suggesting that they are of equal value.

ACTIVITY 9.2

Consider the three elements of evidence-based practice:

- The patient's experiences, values and expectations.
- The external evidence – facts and information from the relevant literature.
- Your nursing expertise – your experience and reflections from practice.

List them in what you think is the correct order of importance, explaining the rationale for the order you have identified.

Check the activity answers at the end of the chapter to see if our thoughts are similar.

When considering the importance of the three elements of evidence-based practice, there is a view that evidence-based practice overemphasises the value of scientific/research evidence (the external evidence) and underplays the role of your nursing expertise which is the result of your personal observations and reflections on your practice (Noorani et al., 2018).

If you refer to your answer for Activity 9.2, did you find it simple to put the three elements of evidence-based practice in order of importance or was it difficult to make a judgement? When trying to rank the elements of evidence-based practice in order of importance, I find it impossible to make a distinction between the value of the scientific/research evidence and nursing expertise. This is because it is our nursing expertise that enables us to know how to deliver care, and as we continue to gain new experiences and increase our knowledge, we develop from a novice nurse to an expert (Benner, 1984). Thus, we develop our nursing expertise by increasing our personal evidence of what is effective in nursing practice. Have you ever watched an expert baker mix and then knead the dough they are going to turn into bread? While the recipe will tell them to add an exact amount of water, an expert baker will know exactly how the dough needs to 'feel'. They will add different amounts of water to achieve this, depending on the individual batch of flour they are using, or the weather, regardless of what the recipe says. An expert baker knows, again by how the dough feels, when it is time to stop kneading and start proving. They are applying their baking expertise, their personal baking evidence. In a similar way, it is nursing expertise, their personal nursing evidence, that enables expert nurses to make **intuitive** and reasoned decisions. While there is no disputing the importance of basing your nursing care on sound, contemporary scientific and research evidence, applying your nursing expertise is just as important. In the same way that an expert baker knows how to mix and treat ingredients to produce a perfect loaf, you apply your nursing expertise to customise an evidence-based plan of care to an individual patient's specific needs.

Reflection is an important aspect of nursing expertise and therefore plays a significant role in evidence-based practice. While we talk about the triad of evidence-based practice, such an approach seems to unnecessarily differentiate between the external evidence and your nursing expertise or, in other words, your personal nursing evidence. In reality, these two elements of the triad are fundamentally intertwined. Such a view is not a new one: nearly twenty years ago Booth (2003) suggested that the evidence in evidence-based practice should not focus on research-derived evidence alone, but should take a wider approach which embodies nursing expertise based on reflective practice. Therefore, Figure 9.2 redraws the usually accepted diagram of evidence-based practice in order to accurately recognise nursing expertise as a form of evidence.

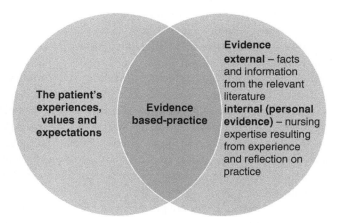

Figure 9.2 Evidence-based practice: redrawing the triad to unite evidence gained from differing approaches

In Figure 9.2, we still have the three elements of evidence-based practice, but the elements previously known as 'the external evidence' and 'your nursing expertise' have been united. There is, however, recognition that these types of evidence arise from different approaches. External evidence is that outside the nurse, the relevant scientific and research-based literature; internal evidence is the personal body of knowledge and experience developed within the nurse as they progress from novice to expert. To split these two into separate spheres does not recognise the importance of combining the scientific and research-based approach with nursing expertise in order to achieve effective, high-quality care. Uniting the two forms of evidence enables the true value of nursing expertise – personal evidence based on learning through reflection – to be recognised.

The approach taken in Figure 9.2 also enables the **concept** of nursing intuition to be demystified.

ACTIVITY 9.3

Using internet search engines, online dictionaries or hard copy versions, or a combination of these, find three definitions of the term 'nursing intuition'. Write a brief note explaining how these definitions help you to understand the term.

Check the activity answers at the end of the chapter to see if our thoughts are similar.

The concept of nursing intuition and its role in clinical practice has been considered for many years. Terms such as gut feeling, pattern recognition, discovering similarities, a mystical power, common sense and **tacit knowledge** are all used when discussing the application of nursing intuition to practice. The usage of some of these terms contribute to the idea that nursing intuition is associated with something mysterious (English, 1993), which does little to develop an understanding of how nurses apply their expertise. Nursing intuition is more than simply a 'gut feeling' or 'pattern recognition' and is not a mystical nursing superpower. It is, however, true that the knowledge derived from nursing intuition may be difficult to **articulate** and share. This is because it is tacit knowledge, generated from personal experience. It is a response based on knowledge gained from reflection on the experience of delivering patient care and, as such, plays an important role in expert nursing practice.

Nursing intuition is what Samantha is describing at the start of the chapter. Her experience of 'just knowing' that a patient was becoming increasingly unwell, even though none of their assessments identified this, was due to her nursing intuition. She was recognising the signs she had seen previously at the start of a patient's deterioration, at the point before this deterioration was being reflected in formal assessments. Her nursing expertise, based on knowledge gained from reflecting on previous experience, was enabling her to instinctively recognise deterioration in a patient, even though she was unable to articulate this.

Samantha's experience raises an important practical point when caring for patients. Even if you can't explain clearly why you are concerned about a patient's condition, in order to follow *The Code* (NMC, 2018), we must at all times act on our concerns. Always make sure that you make others aware of your worries and ensure that the patient remains safe.

USING REFLECTION AS A STARTING POINT FOR RESEARCH QUESTIONS

Research occupies a central role in nursing by assisting nurses to determine the most effective practice and thus improve patient care. Within all nurse education programmes, students are supported to find, read, critique and apply nursing research, enabling them to develop the skills to ensure that their practice will remain contemporary and evidence-based.

Have you ever wondered, however, why nurse researchers choose to investigate the subjects they do? Research often starts 'on the front lines of patient care' as, during our daily interactions with patients, it is not unusual to meet situations that generate questions as to exactly what best practice is. From the simplest to the most complex, questions relating to clinical practice are frequently the starting points for research projects that ultimately determine the best evidence-based practices to ensure high-quality patient care.

ACTIVITY 9.4

Refer to the case study of Rati Patil in Part C. Thinking about what Rati highlights in her reflection, what questions can you identify that could be a starting point for a research project?

Check the activity answers at the end of the chapter to see if our thoughts are similar.

If you speak to many nurses who undertake research, reflection on specific nursing experience is often a trigger for them to decide to undertake a research project. Frequently, the motivation for them to commence research is that they wish to understand an experience more fully and find out what changes could be made in order to improve care. Nursing researchers are real people who function in the same everyday situations as us and ask the same question: 'how can I improve what I am doing?'.

Research investigation often focuses on the nurse researcher's current practice with the aim of making changes to improve care and enable the researcher to make sense of a situation. In other words, research itself can often be a process enabling individuals to reflect on their own practice, with this element of self-reflection even being crucial to some research methodologies. Action research is an example of this, as throughout its application researchers are supported to plan what changes can be made, implement these changes and then reflect once again.

Reflection plays an essential role in many other types of qualitative research, as throughout their studies qualitative researchers not only enquire into the experiences of others, but simultaneously consider their own functioning, as both researchers and practitioners. Reflection, therefore, when used as a tool for promoting actions, analysing how and why things happen and identifying assumptions, becomes a critical component of nursing research and a way to generate knowledge for care based on practice experience.

REFLECTION AS A BRIDGE BETWEEN THEORY AND PRACTICE

ACTIVITY 9.5

Using an online search engine or a library search tool, undertake a search for articles written about the 'theory practice gap in nursing'.

1.   How many articles did your search locate?
2.   What was the date of the earliest published article in your search?

Check the activity answers at the end of the chapter to see if our thoughts are similar.

The gap between theory and practice has been widely documented and considered in the nursing literature for over sixty years. Despite this large body of evidence, newly qualified nurses continue to report experiencing 'transition shock' (Duchscher, 2009) in their first post as a registered nurse. This clearly highlights the gap between the knowledge acquired in a nursing student's professional education and the knowledge they need to cope in practice. Frequently, newly qualified nurses describe their first year as a registered nurse as not only a tough experience, but one involving a large amount of both professional and personal learning and development. Despite successfully completing a nursing programme which includes frequent experiences in nursing practice, once registered, applying previously gained theoretical knowledge to daily nursing practice can still prove difficult. Further to this, as we found in the literature search in Activity 9.5, this is a situation we have been aware of for more than half a century. As it has existed for this length of time, despite numerous research investigations and the introduction of measures to improve the situation, the issue is clearly complex and likely to involve more than just one factor. However, being able to understand the link between the theory taught on a nursing programme and the practical aspects of providing care is vital, and not just an issue of concern for newly registered nurses.

Throughout all stages of a nursing programme, it is important that experience in practice builds on the theory that has already been taught, and that practical nursing experience increases the understanding of the theory. To be able to practise effectively, all nurses need to perceive the **coherence** between theory and practice. We need to understand the link between the two elements of nursing theory and nursing practice, and apply them in our nursing care as a unified whole. This is not simple to achieve and does not magically happen in the final module of a nursing programme or accompany a nursing registration document. Work to achieve this by the end of a nursing programme commences at the very start.

Reflective practice, which includes critical thinking and reflection on experiences, is a method of bridging the gap between theory and practice. In addition to this, it also enables the development of tacit knowledge and the ability to articulate it (Hatlevik, 2012). Thus, the importance of reflective practice is highlighted in its role as a way to ensure high-quality patient care. As shown in Figure 9.3, reflective practice provides us with a bridge between the **abstract** nature of theory and everyday nursing practice.

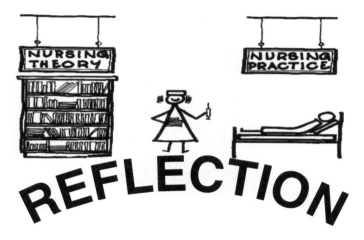

Figure 9.3 Reflection: the bridge between nursing theory and practice

Our reflective skills are **generic**, which means that they are not related to a specific context or theme, and therefore applicable to all areas of nursing practice and nursing subjects. Gaining both practical experience and practical competencies are critical features of the development of professional expertise (Benner, 1984). Applying a reflective approach to this experience to 'make it meaningful' and learn from it is how we develop over time from a novice to an expert practitioner. While it is essential to have scientific knowledge and technical know-how in all aspects of nursing practice, they are not, on their own, sufficient. We need more than this to deliver effective nursing care. To function effectively as a nurse, we need to be able to deliver compassionate care underpinned by theory. Reflection is the bridge that makes the connection.

ACTIVITY 9.6

Read the reflections written by Angus in Part A, Florence in Part B and Rati in Part C. Make a list of the features these three reflections share.

Check the activity answers at the end of the chapter to see if our thoughts are similar.

If you compare a number of reflections written by different individuals, you are likely to see that they contain a number of similar elements. Indeed, if you refer to Chapter 1, we see that we identified 'six essential elements of a good reflection' (see Figure 9.4).

Thus, we should be able to see all of these six elements in every reflection. There does, however, need to be the addition of a further essential element, which surpasses those listed in Figure 9.4.

The vitally important element of any reflection, which will enable the reflection to become a bridge between nursing theory and nursing practice, is that it must consider theory relevant to the experience. Referring to the six essential elements of a good reflection in Figure 9.4, theory is **implicit** in 3, 4 and 5, but to gain the most from every reflection you must make the theory you are considering **explicit**.

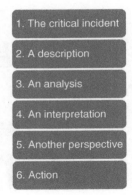

Figure 9.4   The six essential elements of a good reflection

While this may sound obvious, often the easiest part of a reflection to write is the description of what happened. To identify and apply the relevant theory and then to analyse it, is a much more complex academic skill. As you have seen in the reflections contained in this book, analysing the relevant theory takes careful consideration and application of all the critical thinking skills outlined in Chapter 3. Angus in Part A, Florence in Part B and Rati in Part C each make clear their attempts to do this, but they are all still developing their skills. An exemplary example of how to include, apply and analyse theory in a reflection is provided by Gail in Chapter 5. To be able to achieve this takes practice, but in terms of what you gain in nursing expertise and the ability to deliver effective care, there is huge reward.

CONCLUSION

To deliver the best possible care for patients, we need to apply scientific research evidence, nursing experience and understand the patient's experiences, values and expectations. Thus, we need to utilise evidence-based practice. While the application of scientific research evidence is important, combining this with nursing expertise – our personal evidence – is essential. Evidence-based practice has been accused of valuing scientific research evidence more highly than nursing expertise. In reality, however, these two elements of evidence-based practice are so deeply intertwined that they form two parts of one whole. Reflection plays a part in this, as it enables us to make our experience meaningful and to learn from it.

Nursing intuition has been referred to as 'gut feeling' or a 'mystical power'. There is no magic involved in nursing intuition; it develops from reflection on experience and as such plays an important role in expert nursing practice.

The importance of research in nursing is clear and the starting point for research undertaken by nurse researchers is often a reflection. Many research projects evolve from the simple question of 'How can what I am doing be improved?'.

To be able to practise effectively as a nurse – throughout your nursing student programme, and from a newly registered nurse to an experienced nursing expert – it is necessary to link theory with practice. The key to achieving this is reflection as it enables you to see the coherence between the two. Thus, when reflecting in any format, it is vital to consider theory relevant to the experience.

---------------------- GOING FURTHER ----------------------

Benner, P. (1984) *From Novice to Expert*. Menlo Park, CA: Addison-Wesley. This is a seminal text, which remains relevant to practice today in its explanation of how nurses develop from novice to expert and the importance of learning how to nurse, as well as developing knowledge of nursing theory.

Melin-Johansson, C., Palmqvist, R. and Ronnberg, L. (2017) Clinical intuition in the nursing process and decision-making – A mixed-studies review. *Journal of Clinical Nursing*, 26: 3936–49. A thought-provoking article reviewing the data from 16 studies which finds that intuition plays a key role in many of the steps in the nursing process.

Intuition. Go to: www.ausmed.com/cpd/articles/clinical-intuitive-intelligence. A discussion of intuitive intelligence and its value in nursing.

---------------------- ANSWERS TO ACTIVITIES ----------------------

Activity 9.1

Evidence-based practice is the combination of scientific evidence derived from research, individual nursing expertise and the patient's experiences, values and expectations. It is the way that we deliver accountable, professional nursing care. By consciously considering the best evidence we have when making decisions about patient care, in combination with the patient's perspective and our nursing expertise, we can provide the highest quality care possible for the patient.

Activity 9.2

There is no correct answer for this question; your view on this is just as acceptable as mine, and actually the important part of doing this activity is to be able to explain why you put the elements in the order you did. I struggle to answer this question with a simple answer, putting the three elements in a list of reducing value, because I think two of the elements are equal. In my list the elements are ordered:

1.   The patient's experiences, values and expectations.
2.   External evidence *and* your nursing expertise.

This choice of ordering reflects my view that we must always put the patient first in any aspect of their care and treatment, so their experiences, values and expectations must be the first consideration as to whether any care is the best for them – thus, this is my number 1. I then have a tie for my number 2. Ensuring that patient care is based on external evidence is of huge importance, but as I interpret, relate and apply this to each individual patient by using my clinical knowledge and expertise, it becomes impossible to rank one higher than the other.

Activity 9.3

These are the definitions I found:

1.   The ability for knowing or doing without adequate reasons.

(Continued)

2.   A legitimate knowledge in nursing – tacit knowledge.
3.   A mystical power that appears from nowhere.

While I love the third definition of nursing intuition, as it seems to tell me that nursing intuition is our nursing superpower, I don't agree that there is any magical element in intuition. I think that the first definition is partly correct – that nursing intuition is an ability for knowing or doing – but I don't agree that it is without adequate reason. I think just because we might not be able to fully identify the reasons, it doesn't mean that they are not adequate.

Definition two is, I think, the most helpful for my understanding. Nursing intuition is a legitimate form of nursing knowledge, but as it is tacit, it originates from personal experience and is difficult to articulate or share.

Activity 9.4

When I read Rati's reflection, I found six questions that I thought could be a good starting point for a research project. You may well have found more than this. My six questions were:

1.   What information is missed in handover?
2.   How effectively do nursing students communicate with patients living with dementia?
3.   Does the criteria used to identify patients who need a 'special' identify the appropriate patients?
4.   How can nurses be helped to use the emotional aspect of conversations to improve their ability to communicate with patients living with dementia?
5.   What is the risk of not performing your own assessment on patients as soon as they come into your care?
6.   How can communication with patients living with dementia be improved within the acute setting?

The next step to take would be to complete a literature review relating to each of these questions, as it may be that they could be answered by existing literature and research data. If the answers still can't be found, or the answers are too old to be relevant to current practice, the area may well be a good focus for a research project.

Activity 9.5

1.   I used a university library search tool for my search and found that there were 4,029 items relevant to my search. Looking through the items identified (briefly), it did seem that most of them were relevant to the topic, so from this I think that it is possible to say that there is a great deal of consideration of this topic in the relevant nursing literature.
2.   Looking to see the date range of the items (you can do this by reordering the search to 'oldest first', usually by clicking on the button at the top of your search list, which will probably say 'relevance' at the moment), the oldest item was written in 1955. From this information I think that we can add to our previous conclusion and say that not only is there a great deal of literature relating to the theory–practice gap, but the topic has been considered for over more than sixty years.

Activity 9.6

My list includes two features – you may have found more.

1. Apply a model of reflection – these are different, but are all frequently used reflective models that help to structure the writing.
2. Make reference to relevant theory: some consider more theory than others, but this is a fundamentally important element of any reflection; it must consider the theory relevant to the experience being reflected on.

GLOSSARY

abstract   Existing in thought or as an idea, but not having a physical or concrete existence.

articulate   The ability to talk about an issue fluently and coherently.

coherence   The quality of being logical and consistent, forming a unified whole.

concept   An abstract idea.

explicit   Stated clearly and in detail.

facilitates   Makes an action or a process easier.

generic   Not specific; can be applied to different situations.

implicit   Suggested but not directly expressed.

intuitive   Instinctive, based on what one feels to be true even without conscious reasoning.

tacit knowledge   Knowledge generated from personal experience that is instinctive.

triad of evidence-based practice   This term is used to refer to the three elements of evidence-based practice: evidence (facts and information from the relevant literature), your nursing expertise, and the patient's experiences, values and expectations.

REFERENCES

Benner, P. (1984) *From Novice to Expert*. Menlo Park, CA: Addison-Wesley.

Booth, A. (2003) Where systems meet services: towards evidence based information practice. *Vine*, 33(2): 65–71.

Duchscher, J. (2009) Transition shock: the initial stage of role adaptation for newly graduated registered nurses. *Journal of Advanced Nursing*, 65: 1103–13.

English, I. (1993) Intuition as a function of the expert nurse: a critique of Benner's novice to expert model. *Journal of Advanced Nursing*, 18: 387–93.

Hatlevik, I. (2012) The theory-practice relationship: reflective skills and theoretical knowledge as key factors in bridging the gap between theory and practice in initial nursing education. *Journal of Advanced Nursing*, 68(4): 868–77.

Nursing and Midwifery Council (NMC) (2018) *The Code*. London, NMC.

Noorani, T., Karlsson, M. and Borkman T. (2018) Deep experiential knowledge: reflections from mutual aid groups for evidence-based practice. *Evidence & Policy: A Journal of Research, Debate and Practice*, 15(2): 217–34.

Thorpe, G. and Delves-Yates, C. (2018) Chapter 3, Core Academic Skills. In C. Delves-Yates (ed.) *Essentials of Nursing Practice* (2nd edn), pp. 35–52. London: SAGE.

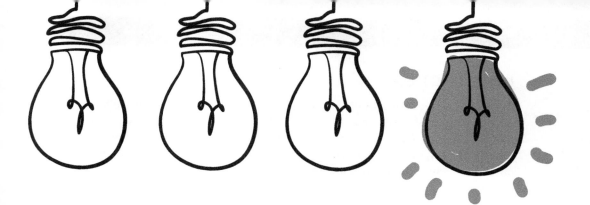

SO MANY MODELS . . .

CATHERINE DELVES-YATES

> A reflective model, a reflective framework or a reflective tool? What do I call it?
>
> **Mo Bailey-Winston, registered nurse, adult field**

> I have done lots of reflections using lots of different models. I can see that they help me to focus my thinking, but now I want to be more adventurous! Can I reflect without using a model?
>
> **Jasper Betty, nursing student, learning disability field**

INTRODUCTION

As Mo asks at the very start of the chapter – what should we call them? What we will refer to as 'models' in this chapter are also known as frameworks of reflection, reflective tools or even reflective cycles. To answer Mo's question, generally the terms are used interchangeably, so you can use any of them, but be consistent with the term you use, as otherwise it will become confusing for anyone reading what you write.

Using a model when reflecting helps you to focus on learning from experience, develop your self-awareness and avoid simply retelling what happened. Models give your writing a structure, increase the **analytical** depth and guide you through the process of reflection. There is, however, no 'best' or 'right' model; you need to choose the one that feels most comfortable for you and assists you to learn from your experience. Or, as Jasper suggests and we will discuss later, you might decide you want to reflect without the aid of a model.

In this chapter, we are going to develop further the knowledge of models you have gained from previous chapters, introducing three more models which are frequently applied and found helpful in the process of reflection. We are also going to consider how you can customise a model to meet your own individual requirements, and discuss the value of reflecting without applying a model.

──────────────── CHAPTER AIMS ────────────────

This chapter will enable you to:

- appreciate the characteristics common to all models of reflection;
- realise that there is no one best model of reflection;
- understand how to apply Gibbs's (1988) model to your reflections;
- become familiar with the REFLECT model and know how to use it to structure a reflection;
- understand the approach taken by Johns's (1995) model of structured reflection and the specific experience to which it is applicable;
- appreciate the positives and negatives of free-form reflection.

INTRODUCING FURTHER REFLECTIVE MODELS

ACTIVITY 10.1

- Before reading any further, make a list of what you feel are the benefits of using a model of reflection.

Check the activity answers at the end of the chapter to see if our thoughts are similar.

All models of reflection are guides that enable you to analyse an experience in a systematic fashion in order to promote improvements in your care. Using a model will assist you to understand your own thinking, relate new knowledge to previous understanding and identify new strategies to improve your practice.

All models are based on the four key **concepts** of reflection identified in Figure 10.1, which is why many models look similar to each other.

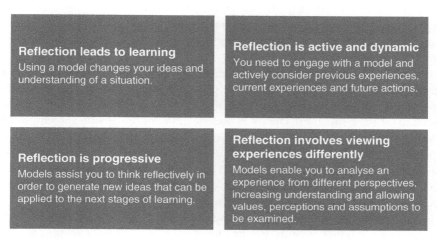

Reflection leads to learning
Using a model changes your ideas and understanding of a situation.

Reflection is active and dynamic
You need to engage with a model and actively consider previous experiences, current experiences and future actions.

Reflection is progressive
Models assist you to think reflectively in order to generate new ideas that can be applied to the next stages of learning.

Reflection involves viewing experiences differently
Models enable you to analyse an experience from different perspectives, increasing understanding and allowing values, perceptions and assumptions to be examined.

Figure 10.1   Four key concepts

As we said at the start of the chapter, sometimes models are referred to as reflective cycles. This is because reflection is a progressive process; what you learn from one stage of your reflection is applied to the next. Thus, many models, as you will see in the models of Gibbs (1988) and Johns (1995), are presented in the form of a cycle. Other models, such as Borton's (1970), which Angus used in his reflection in Part A, are **linear**. How a model is presented, however, doesn't alter the need to apply what you learn from one stage of your reflection to the next. This clearly demonstrates that reflection is a process which, once started, becomes ongoing.

The ongoing nature of reflection is clearly highlighted by Johns (2017) in his consideration of the process we undergo when developing ourselves from 'doing reflection' to 'being reflective'. This process is shown at the start of this book in Figure 1.1 on p. 8. You will be very familiar with this figure, as we have referred to it in a number of previous chapters, but it is important to consider it again here because it underpins what we wish to achieve. 'Being reflective' is the state we are working towards, but unlike being awarded a degree certificate, where there is a final end point to your learning, to truly attain the state of 'being reflective' we need to keep applying and reflecting on all we have experienced and learnt.

Returning to the point of similarity between models, essentially they are similar because they function in the same way. Models help you to think in a reflective manner in order to answer 'the five Whats?' as shown in Figure 10.2, and therefore learn from your experience.

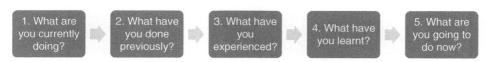

1. What are you currently doing? → 2. What have you done previously? → 3. What have you experienced? → 4. What have you learnt? → 5. What are you going to do now?

Figure 10.2   The five Whats?

THERE IS NO 'RIGHT' MODEL

A good way to think of what we are doing when we are reflecting is that we are 'consciously exploring an experience'. As we have said throughout many of the previous chapters, in order to learn from experience, you need to reflect on it. Using a model as a learning tool in order to do this is an effective approach. Models are particularly useful as they prompt you to move away from undertaking actions in an 'auto-pilot' approach by encouraging you to ask questions and challenge your assumptions.

There are numerous models of reflection; it is up to you to choose whichever model you feel best assists your learning. Further to this, you may decide not to limit yourself to just using one model for all your reflections, as you might want to apply different models to differing situations. Once you become more confident with applying models, as Jasper was at the start of the chapter, you too may want to be more adventurous. Jasper was interested in reflecting without using a model, but a good exercise to undertake before doing this is to develop a model of your own. You can do this by combining two (or more) models you are familiar with to devise the individual framework you feel best supports your reflective thinking and analysis of your experience.

In this textbook so far, in Part A we considered Borton's (1970) model of reflection and outlined a number of hints and tips for using this. We have also seen the NMC (2018) framework being used by Florence in Part B, and outlined the similarities between this model and Borton's. In Part C, Rati applied Gibbs's (1988) model to her reflection, so we are now going to consider this model in more detail.

GIBBS'S (1988) REFLECTIVE CYCLE

Gibbs's (1988) reflective cycle is probably one of the most frequently used models of reflection. It tends to be the first model many nurse education programmes encourage students to use, because it leads you through the different stages very clearly and simply helps make meaning from experience.

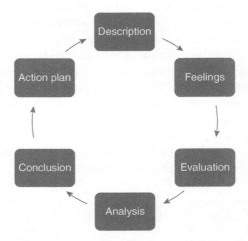

Figure 10.3   Gibbs's (1988) reflective cycle

Gibbs's model can be applied to reflection on any type of experience. It is, however, often recommended to assist learning from everyday situations because its cyclic nature lends itself particularly well to repeated experiences. Such an approach enables you to learn from things that either went well or didn't go so well, then make plans for future actions based on this learning.

Gibbs's model encourages you to systematically consider your experience by presenting six stages, with key questions to consider in each stage. The model starts by asking for a clear description of the experience, and then leads you through the reflection and the resulting learning, which is finally applied in a plan of what you would do if the situation arose again. The stages of the model are presented in Figure 10.3.

The key questions you need to consider in each stage of Gibbs's model (see Table 10.1) are especially helpful for those new to reflection, as they are a sound guide and prompt you to consider the issues relevant to each stage.

Table 10.1 Key questions to consider in each stage of Gibbs's (1988) model

Stage of Gibbs's (1988) model	Questions to prompt your reflective thinking
Description In this stage, the aim is to describe the experience in detail, so make sure that you clearly identify exactly what happened.	• What happened? • When did it happen? • Where did it happen? • Why were you there? • Who was present? • What did you do? • What did other people do? • What did you want to happen? • What was the result of the situation?
Feelings In this stage, the aim is to explore the feelings and/or thoughts that you had during the experience. Make sure that you identify how they may have an effect on the experience.	• What were you feeling before the experience? • What were you feeling during the experience? • What were you feeling after the experience? • What do you think other people were feeling about the experience at the time it happened? • What do you think other people feel about the experience now? • What were you thinking before the experience? • What were you thinking during the experience? • What do you think about the experience now?

(Continued)

Table 10.1   (Continued)

Stage of Gibbs's (1988) model	Questions to prompt your reflective thinking

Evaluation
 	
In this stage, the aim is to evaluate what worked well and what didn't work in the experience. While it might be difficult, make sure that you are as **objective** and honest as possible.
 	
Remember to focus on both the things that went well and the things that didn't go well, as even in the best or worst experiences, nothing is either exclusively positive or negative.
 	
Remember to support any judgements you make with relevant evidence (reference to theory and/or literature).
	• What was good about the experience?
	• What was bad about the experience?
	• What went well?
	• What could have gone better?
	• Were there things that were:
	  o difficult?
	  o interesting?
	  o surprising?
	  o upsetting?
	• What was your contribution to the experience (positive and/or negative)?
	• What did others contribute to the situation (positive and/or negative)?
	• What judgement can you come to about the experience and any possible consequences?

Analysis In this stage, the aim is to make sense of what happened and make the experience meaningful. In its simplest form, analysis is asking the question 'why?', so make sure that you consider why aspects of the experience went well or badly. This is another stage in the model where it is important to include the evidence for your statements, so support all of your comments with references to theory and/or literature.	• Why did things go well? • Why didn't things go well? • What knowledge do you have that can help you to understand the experience? • What theory can help you to understand the experience? • How do your previous experiences relate to this one? • How did your participation in the experience affect the outcome? • What sense can you make of the experience?

Conclusion
 	
In this stage, the aim is to come to conclusions about what happened. Make sure that you summarise your learning and identify how you would change your actions to improve the outcome in the future.
 	
As in all conclusions, don't introduce any new material here; focus only on what you have discussed previously.
	• What did you learn from this experience?
	• What else could you have done?
	• How could this experience have been made positive for all of those involved?
	• What skills do you need to develop?
	• What
	  o insights
	  o thoughts
	  o conclusions
	relating specifically to your actions in this experience have you gained?

Action plan In this stage, the aim is to plan what you would do in a similar experience in the future. This might include identifying how you will help yourself to act differently. To change your behaviour can be very difficult, so you may need to think of strategies you can use to ensure that you don't repeat previous actions.	• If the experience happened again, what would you do differently? • How will you develop the skills you require? • How can you ensure that you can act differently next time?

ACTIVITY 10.2

Read the reflection written by Rati using Gibbs's (1988) model in Part C.

- Could Rati have included any of the key questions in Table 10.1 in her reflection to make it more effective?

Check the activity answers at the end of the chapter to see if our thoughts are similar.

Working carefully through the stages of Gibbs's (1988) model and answering the key questions will enable you to produce an effective reflection. This model is a particularly useful one to apply if you are reflecting for a formal reason, such as for an academic assignment, because the key questions will help you to achieve the required **learning outcomes** for your assessment. One of the major challenges, however, is being able to answer all the questions if the word allowance for your assignment is small.

THE REFLECT MODEL

It is highly appropriate to consider the REFLECT model (Barksby et al., 2015) after Gibbs (1988), because REFLECT is a modification of Gibbs's model. REFLECT has been specifically developed in order to create a simple-to-use and easy-to-remember model. If you

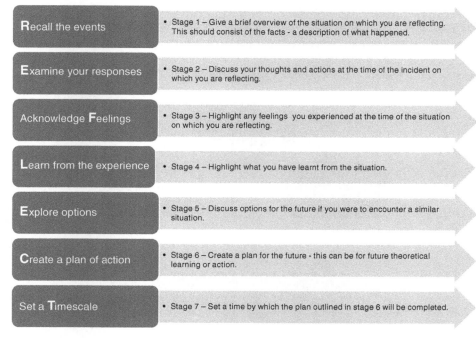

Figure 10.4   The REFLECT model

Source: Barksby et al. (2015) A new model of reflection for clinical practice, *Nursing Practice Review*. Reproduced by kind permission of Justine Barksby.

look at REFLECT, it is clear that it is an adaptation of Gibbs's model because the stages are very similar. The clever part of REFLECT is that it has been created as a **mnemonic** which can be easily remembered. Such an approach was taken in order to enable those using REFLECT to focus on considering the experience they are reflecting on, rather than remembering the model.

Figure 10.4 shows the steps in the model and the areas to focus on during each of these.

Due to the REFLECT model being based on Gibbs's (1988) model, the questions identified in Table 10.1 for the six stages of Gibbs's model, with some minor alterations, could be applied to the first six steps of REFLECT. For the seventh stage of REFLECT – 'timescale' – the guidance already provided does not need any further explanation.

ACTIVITY 10.3

- How would you alter the questions in Table 10.1 so that they would apply to REFLECT?

Check the activity answers at the end of the chapter to see if our thoughts are similar.

JOHNS'S (1995) MODEL OF STRUCTURED REFLECTION

The final model we are going to consider is Johns's (1995). This model was specifically developed for use in nursing, based on **seminal work** by Carper (1978). Johns's model takes a more complex approach to reflection in the exploration of the areas of **aesthetics**, personal knowing, ethics and **empirics**, and then applies this deliberation to assist you to consider how this has changed and improved your practice. Although this model can be used for everyday situations, it is particularly helpful if you are reflecting on and analysing complex decisions. Johns's model has five phases, presented in a cyclical fashion (see Figure 10.5).

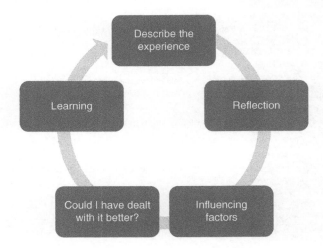

Figure 10.5   Johns's (1995) model of structured reflection

Source: Johns (1995) Framing learning through reflection within Carper's fundamental ways of knowing in nursing. *Journal of Advanced Nursing.* Reproduced by kind permission of John Wiley & Sons.

In his model, Johns suggests that when you reflect it is important to:

- 'look inwards' in order to consider your own thoughts and feelings;
- 'look outwards' in order to consider the experience, whether your actions were ethical and any external factors that influenced you.

Similarly to the other models we have considered, there are a number of 'cue questions' that assist you to do this in each phase of the model. These are presented in Table 10.2.

Johns (1995) also suggests that involving another person to support you in your reflection – for example, your practice supervisor or manager – will result in your learning being more effective than if you reflect alone.

Table 10.2 Cue questions for Johns's (1995) model of structured reflection

Phase of Johns's (1995) model of structured reflection	Cue questions
Describe the experience	Clearly describe the experience, including all of the significant factors involved.
Reflection	What were you trying to achieve?
	What were the consequences of your actions?
	How did you feel about this experience as it was happening?
	Why did you feel like this?
	How did any other people involved in the experience feel about the situation?
Influencing factors	What factors (e.g. internal factors, your own knowledge, external factors) affected your actions and decision making?
Could I have dealt with it better?	What other choices did you have? Could you have acted in another way?
	Did you act for the best?
	What would the consequences of those other actions have been for you and for others?
Learning	What will change because of this experience?
	How do you now feel about the experience?
	How has this experience changed your ways of knowing in respect of:
	• Empirics (scientific/research) knowledge?
	• Ethical (moral) knowledge?
	• Personal (self-awareness) knowledge?
	• Aesthetic (the art of what we do) knowledge?

If you compare the cue questions from Johns's (1995) model to the questions for Gibbs's (1988) model, I think it is possible to understand why Gibbs's model is frequently recommended for those starting to develop their reflective skills. Gibbs's model provides greater guidance and a simpler approach. However, as mentioned before, Johns's (1995) model is a very good one to apply if you want to reflect on a complex decision. The consideration of empirics, ethics and aesthetics is something not highlighted by other models, and as you increase your understanding of reflection, this presents an excellent way to develop your knowledge further.

ACTIVITY 10.4

Consider the three models we have discussed in detail in this chapter – Gibbs's (1988) model, REFLECT and Johns's (1995) model of structured reflection.

- Which one will you choose for your next reflection? Provide a rationale for your answer.

Check the activity answers at the end of the chapter to see if our thoughts are similar.

BREAKING FREE FROM MODELS

At the start of the chapter, Jasper asked whether it is possible to reflect without using a model. It most certainly is. When you are producing a reflection you can choose either to apply a structured model or use a free-form approach. Free-form, or unstructured reflection, is when we don't apply a model to reflect on an experience.

There is, however, a step between using a **validated** model and the liberated approach of free-form reflection. This is actually the approach that Barksby et al. (2015) undertook when they developed REFLECT. As we have discussed, they adapted Gibbs's (1988) model to develop a new model of their own. If you wish to alter how you reflect, but cannot find a model that provides what you are looking for, you can, like Barksby et al. (2015), adapt an existing model, or even combine elements of two or more reflective models that have elements that assist you to reflect. So, for example, in my answer to Activity 10.4, I said that I use both Gibbs's and Johns's models, as I find that these models enable me to think deeply about aspects of my experience that I feel are important. I could, therefore, combine the elements I find most effective in these models and produce my own personal model to support my reflections. This may well take considerable time, and the new model would need to be tested, evaluated and probably adapted, but the end result could be that my model becomes very popular.

If, however, rather than taking this approach you want to join Jasper in trying free-form reflection, there are a few points to consider first.

Free-form reflecting is a good approach if, rather than following the structure of a model, you just want to start thinking and see where this takes you. Due to this issue, I would suggest that submitting a free-form reflection for an academic assignment is a very risky approach to take, as you may well not address the issues required in a formal assessment. That is not to say, however, that the exercise would not be without value for your personal learning; it just might not gain you many marks in a formal assessment.

In free-form reflection, you can just allow the words to flow. If you are experienced at reflection it is likely that you may, even subconsciously, follow the format of a reflective model, or perhaps your thoughts will be totally unconstrained. The value of free-form reflection is that you don't limit yourself to answer a particular set of predefined questions. It is likely that the end result will be a very personal reflection. When producing a personal reflection, rather than a more formal reflection for an assignment, for example, you can be as unconstrained as you wish, although you do need to remember that personal reflections in whatever shape or form still need to uphold the definition of reflection, as otherwise they are just writing and not reflections. Remember, what you should end up with is the conscious consideration of your thoughts and actions. While there are some issues you need to consider before undertaking free-form reflection, there are benefits. The positive and negative points to consider when undertaking free-form reflection are presented in Figure 10.6.

You can exlore different elements of your experience and thoughts as they appear to you.	It would be risky to use this approach to reflection for an assignment, as you may not address the areas required.
There is no one right way.	It is easy to switch between reflecting
You can let your thoughts run free!	and just writing, so constantly ensure that what you are doing upholds the definition of reflection.
You can start your reflection however you wish, with your thoughts, your learning or the feelings that prompted you to reflect.	You can end up 'stuck' with a thought, as you do not have a structure to develop it.
Your thoughts do not have to be restricted to fit into a model.	If you are not rigorous in the questions you ask yourself, you may miss important areas of thinking which would aid your learning.
You can ask yourself questions which do not fit into a model.	

Figure 10.6   Points to consider when undertaking free-form reflection

CONCLUSION

No matter whether a model is presented as a cycle or in a straight line, they all share a number of characteristics as they are based on the same key concepts. There is no 'right' model of reflection. It is up to you to choose a model that works best for you and is appropriate for the reason you are undertaking the reflection.

For many nursing students, Gibbs's (1988) model is one they are encouraged to use, as it provides comprehensive guidance as how to reflect effectively. An adaptation of Gibbs's model is REFLECT, which has been specifically designed to be easy to remember and apply. A further model, which is frequently used by students, especially to reflect on experiences where complex decisions were taken, is Johns's (1995) model, which enables clear consideration of the ethical aspects of a situation. It is also possible to develop a model of your own or to customise an existing model.

If you wish to break free from models, free-form reflection may be something to try. If you do decide, however, to reflect free-form, it is important to consider both the positives and the negatives of this approach. Most importantly, you would need to be extremely certain that you achieve the required learning outcomes for an assignment if you chose to adopt this approach in a formal assessment.

Once we start out on a journey to become a reflective practitioner, reflection becomes an ongoing cyclical process. We need always to work towards 'being reflective', and to keep 'being reflective', we have to keep reflecting.

GOING FURTHER

Coward, M. (2011) Does the use of reflective models restrict critical thinking and therefore learning in nurse education? What have we done? *Nurse Education Today*, 31: 883–6. An interesting article which investigates the author's view that applying a model in a reflection actually serves to restrict thinking rather than develop it.

Gibbs, G. (1988). *Learning by Doing: A Guide to Teaching and Learning Methods*. Further Education Unit. Oxford Polytechnic: Oxford. The seminal text, including Gibbs's model, was the result of a collaborative project between Graham Gibbs of Oxford Polytechnic, and Bob Farmer and Diana Eastcott of Birmingham Polytechnic (now Birmingham City University).

Models. Go to: https://lifelonglearningwithot.wordpress.com/2016/05/02/different-models-of-reflection-using-them-to-help-me-reflect/. A guide to a range of models of reflection suggesting the situation in which it is appropriate to apply each model.

ANSWERS TO ACTIVITIES

Activity 10.1

The benefits of using a model of reflection are:

* You are given a clear structure to follow.
* You are provided with 'trigger questions' to focus your thinking.
* Working through the stages of the model, rather than trying to focus on all aspects of your experience at once, stops you from feeling so overwhelmed.
* The process has a clear start and an end.
* You can review examples of how others have applied the model, which can assist you to understand how to reflect effectively.

Activity 10.2

Table 10.3   Rati's reflection based on Gibbs's (1988) model

Questions to prompt your reflective thinking when using Gibbs's (1988) model in Rati's reflection (✓ = question answered; X = question not answered)

While the comments below indicate how many of the questions Rati answered, it is important to remember that her reflection was less than 1,000 words in length, which makes it challenging to address all the questions.

Description

* What happened? ✓
* When did it happen? ✓
* Where did it happen? ✓

- Why were you there? ✓
- Who was present? ✓
- What did you do? ✓
- What did other people do? ✓
- What did you want to happen? X
- What was the result of the situation? ✓

Rati's description answered all these questions apart from saying what she wanted to happen. This would have been a good thing to include, as it would have enabled her to evaluate (in the later stage) whether this was appropriate.

Feelings

- What were you feeling before the experience? X
- What were you feeling during the experience? ✓
- What were you feeling after the experience? X – not explicit
- What do you think other people were feeling about the experience at the time it happened? X
- What do you think other people feel about the experience now? X
- What were you thinking before the experience? X
- What were you thinking during the experience? X – not explicit
- What do you think about the experience now? X – not explicit

In this stage, Rati only concentrated on how she was feeling during the experience. It is possible that some of her thoughts are implicit, but her reflection would have been improved by explicitly identifying what she was thinking as well as what she was feeling, plus considering the feelings of others. This needed to be before, during and after the experience.

Evaluation

- What was good about the experience? ✓
- What was bad about the experience? X – not explicit
- What went well? ✓
- What could have gone better? X – not explicit
- Were there things that were:
  - difficult? X – not explicit
  - interesting? X – not explicit
  - surprising? X – not explicit
  - upsetting? X – not explicit
- What was your contribution to the experience (positive and/or negative)? ✓
- What did others contribute to the situation (positive and/or negative)? X
- What judgement can you come to about the experience and any possible consequences? ✓

In this stage, Rati did consider a number of the questions, but she needed to be more explicit, think in greater detail about what happened, about the contribution of others to the experience and identify what could have gone better.

Analysis

- Why did things go well? ✓
- Why didn't things go well? ✓

(Continued)

Table 10.3 (Continued)

- What knowledge do you have that can help you to understand the experience? ✓
- What theory can help you to understand the experience? X
- How do your previous experiences relate to this one? ✓
- How did your participation in the experience affect the outcome? ✓
- What sense can you make of the experience? ✓

Rati answered lots of the questions in this stage, but, as is so often the case, she missed the opportunity to relate sufficient theory to her practice. As we have discussed in previous chapters, this is so important in reflections as it enables you to link what you do to the relevant theory. I would like to have seen Rati include theory relating to communication in this stage.

Conclusion

- What did you learn from this experience? ✓
- What else could you have done? ✓
- How could this experience have been made positive for all of those involved? X
- What skills do you need to develop? X - not explicit
- What
    - ○ insights
    - ○ thoughts
    - ○ conclusions

relating specifically to your actions in this experience have you gained? ✓

In this stage, Rati again answered many of the questions, but needed to think about the experience from the perspective of others and could have been more explicit in some of her answers.

Action plan

- If the experience happened again, what would you do differently? ✓
- How will you develop the skills you require? ✓
- How can you ensure that you can act differently next time? X – not explicit

Rati's action plan was very good, if she had included how she would have ensured she would act differently next time, it would have been perfect.

Activity 10.3

Table 10.4 Key questions to consider in each stage of REFLECT

Stage of REFLECT	Questions to prompt your reflective thinking
Recall the events. Give a brief overview of the situation on which you are reflecting. This should consist of the facts - a description of what happened.	• What happened? • When did it happen? • Where did it happen? • Why were you there? • Who was present? • What did you do? • What did other people do? • What did you want to happen? • What was the result of the situation?

Stage of REFLECT	Questions to prompt your reflective thinking
Examine your responses.	• What were you thinking during the experience?
Discuss your thoughts and actions at the time of the incident on which you are reflecting.	• Why did you act in the way you did?
Feelings: these need to be examined.	• What were you feeling during the experience?
Highlight any feelings you experienced at the time of the situation on which you are reflecting.	• What do you think other people were feeling about the experience at the time it happened?
Learn from the experience.	• What was good about the experience?
Highlight what you have learnt from the situation.	• What was bad about the experience?
	• What went well?
It is important to include the evidence for your statements in this stage, so support all your comments with references to theory and/or literature.	• What could have gone better?
	• Were there things that were
	o difficult?
	o interesting?
	o surprising?
	o upsetting?
	• What was your contribution to the experience (positive and/or negative)?
	• What did others contribute to the situation (positive and/or negative)?
	• What judgement can you come to about the experience and any possible consequences?
	• Why did things go well?
	• Why didn't things go well?
	• What knowledge do you have that can help you to understand the experience?
	• What theory can help you to understand the experience?
	• How do your previous experiences relate to this one?
	• How did your participation in the experience affect the outcome?
	• What sense can you make of the experience?
	• What did you learn from this experience?
Explore options.	• What else could you have done?
Discuss options for the future if you were to encounter a similar situation.	• How could this experience have been made positive for all of those involved?
	• What skills do you need to develop?
	• What
	o insights
	o thoughts
	o conclusions
	• relating specifically to your actions in this experience have you gained?

(Continued)

Table 10.4   (Continued)

Stage of REFLECT	Questions to prompt your reflective thinking
Create a plan of action. Create a plan for the future – this can be for future theoretical learning or action.	• If the experience happened again, what would you do differently? • How will you develop the skills you require? • How can you ensure that you can act differently next time?
Timescale: this needs to be set. Set a time by which the plan outlined in the previous stage will be completed.	• Identify a date for the completion of all of the actions you are going to undertake.

Activity 10.4

There is no right or wrong answer for this activity – we will all make a choice based on our personal views. Depending on what happens in the next experience I reflect on, I will be using either Gibbs's model (if the experience is an everyday one) or Johns's (if the experience is more complex and I wish to focus on the decision(s) I made). I chose to apply these models because I think that they are the ones that best help me to reflect and learn from experiences. I like the questions for Gibbs's model, as they help me to appreciate a wide range of factors in my experience and I like that Johns's model encourages me to focus on ethical and aesthetic aspects, so I can consider my morals and the art underpinning my actions.

GLOSSARY

aesthetics   A set of principles considering artistry – the 'art' of nursing.

analytical   Examining all aspects using logical reasoning.

concepts   Ideas.

empirics   Scientific or research-based approach.

learning outcomes   What students will know or be able to do when they have completed a course or programme.

linear   Arranged in a straight or nearly straight line.

mnemonic   A system, such as a word, which assists in remembering something.

objective   Not influenced by personal feelings or opinions, but based on evidence.

seminal work   A scholarly article that initially presented an idea of great importance.

validated   Of proven accuracy.

REFERENCES

Barksby, J., Butcher, N. and Whysall, A. (2015) A new model of reflection for clinical practice. *Nursing Times*, 111(34/5): 34–5.

Borton, T. (1970) *Reach, Touch and Teach*. London: Hutchinson.

Carper, B. (1978) Fundamental patterns of knowing in nursing. *Advances in Nursing Science*. 1(1): 13–23.

Gibbs, G. (1988) *Learning by Doing: A Guide to Teaching and Learning Methods*. Further Education Unit, Oxford Polytechnic, Oxford.

Johns, C. (1995) Framing learning through reflection within Carper's fundamental ways of knowing in nursing. *Journal of Advanced Nursing*, 22(2): 226–34.

Johns, C. (2017) *Becoming a Reflective Practitioner*. Chichester: Wiley-Blackwell.

Nursing and Midwifery Council (NMC) (2018) *The Code*. London: NMC.

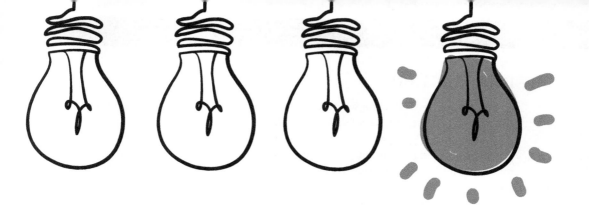

THEORY, PHILOSOPHY AND CRITIQUES

11

CATHERINE DELVES-YATES

> I have just written a reflection for my revalidation! The thinking made my head hurt – what I would like to know is where does the idea of reflection come from?
>
> **Charlie Allen, registered nurse, mental health field**

> Is it really all good? Everything I read about reflection is very positive. Can that really be the case?
>
> **Oscar H. Riley, nursing student, child field**

INTRODUCTION

To be effective in a reflection we need to think very deeply about the focus of our reflective writing, which, as Charlie says at the start of the chapter, can most certainly make your head hurt. It is, however, important to ensure that we think deeply, as otherwise we will not be gaining maximum benefit from our endeavours. Oscar, in his question, also highlights an important issue. While, as we have discussed in previous chapters, there are many benefits of reflection, there are also challenges and limitations. These challenges and limitations are not just in relation to our individual reflections, but also in respect of the role that the knowledge and evidence gained from reflection plays within the future development of nursing.

In this final chapter, we will focus on understanding the theory and philosophy of reflection practice. In doing this, we will consider the origin of the **concept** of reflection and deliberate on potential future development. In essence, we are going to look back to the past and then on to the future. As we discussed in Chapter 4, reflection is the art of looking backwards in order to see how you can apply the learning from your experience to the future, otherwise known as the Janus effect. In this final chapter, we are going to apply this approach to our consideration of the theory, philosophy and critiques of reflection.

─────────────── CHAPTER AIMS ───────────────

This chapter will enable you to:

- understand the theory of reflection;
- appreciate the philosophical perspective of reflective practice;
- realise that reflection started as a radical approach to learning;
- consider the fundamental role that emotion plays in learning;
- become aware of the challenges and limitations of reflection.

THE THEORY AND PHILOSOPHY UNDERPINNING REFLECTION

ACTIVITY 11.1

- Before reading further, write down what you would say were the differences between theory and philosophy.

Check the activity answers at the end of the chapter to see if our thoughts are similar.

The origins of the term 'reflection' are in the Latin term *reflectere*, meaning 'to bend back'. This is what happens to light when it is shone on a mirror, enabling something to be revealed that was previously unknown. This translates directly to the process we call 'reflection', which enables us to view what was previously unknown to us. When we reflect, we are enabled to view our actions, thoughts, values and attitudes, rather than an image in a mirror. The reflection we undertake is a process that creates greater understanding of ourselves based upon our experience and **facilitates** us to apply this new understanding in future actions.

The process of reflection has been viewed as creating our own reality by making sense of our experiences. This thought can be related to a number of spiritual teachings, as shown in Figure 11.1.

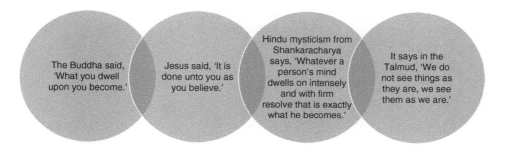

Figure 11.1   A spiritual perspective

From a spiritual perspective, reflection, in the form of serious thought or consideration, contemplation, pondering, meditation or musing, is a tool of growth. The approach we have been taking in the textbook, however, is to consider reflection as a method of assessing and critically evaluating our thoughts and actions in order to learn and develop professionally. There are clear parallels between the two approaches, and thus when we evaluate our thoughts, feelings, beliefs, perceptions and actions within reflective practice, we are not only considering our professional perspective, but also a far more personal one. Our development from reflection is not just professional, but being assisted to view our thoughts, feelings, beliefs and perceptions also facilitates personal growth. Furthermore, spiritual reflection is defined as 'a state of mind', which is also what we are aiming for in our approach. To achieve all these benefits, however, reflection needs to be an ongoing event, not a one-off. As we have discussed in previous chapters, we are aiming to achieve 'being reflective' rather than 'doing reflection' (Johns, 2017).

In its simplest form, the theory underpinning reflection is that by thinking about what you did and what happened, you are able to decide what you would do differently next time. Thus, reflection is a development of the theory of learning from experience, otherwise known as experiential learning. The process of experiential learning is based on the idea that our views, thoughts, ideas, attitudes and values are not permanent and unchangeable, but are constantly modified by experience. Thus, we are in a continuous process of personal learning, which constantly alters our views.

As identified in Figure 11.2, theory relating to experiential learning and reflection has been influenced by a number of individuals over many years.

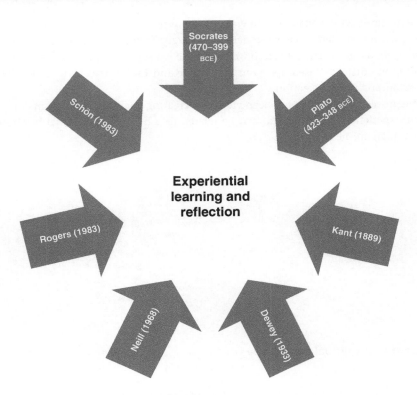

Figure 11.2   Individuals influential in the development of reflection

The theory and philosophy underpinning reflection is not new. It is possible to identify the concept of reflection in the work of the philosophers Socrates and his student Plato more than 2,000 years ago, and in the writing of Kant in the late 1880s. Socrates, a Greek philosopher who has been credited as one of the founders of Western philosophy, is particularly important in the development of reflection. He urged his students to apply a method of 'Socratic questioning' to their thinking, which was designed to help them to develop their thoughts. Socratic questioning enabled students to identify issues and problems, uncover assumptions, analyse concepts and to distinguish what was known from what wasn't. If we keep this approach in mind while reviewing the definitions of reflection in Chapter 1, it is easy to identify a clear relationship between Socratic questioning and reflective practice.

From the perspective of applying reflection to professional issues, however, the work of Dewey (1933) and later Schön (1983, 1987) are arguably the most influential.

John Dewey (1933), in his seminal text *How We Think*, made a lasting impact on teaching and learning, and was one of the first people to write about the relationship between experience, action and reflection. Later, in the 1930s to 1960s, similar ideas were applied to theories of human learning and development, most notably by Kurt Lewin and Jean Piaget, but by others too. Further developments to the theory of experiential learning followed with work since the 1970s frequently focusing on its application to practice – for example, in the work of David Kolb (1984) and Graham Gibbs (1988). You are very likely to be familiar with these names from their reflective models.

It was the educational theorist Donald Schön in 1983, however, who first proposed how professionals could use reflective thinking as a tool to improve their practice. Schön (1983, 1987) put forward the argument that the 'textbook based learning' being used to teach professionals, such as nurses, was not providing all the knowledge they required to practise effectively. Schön (1987, p. 121) states: 'The case is not "in the book"'. What he means by this is that the knowledge we require to deliver care needs to be based on more than pure theory alone.

At this point, we need to appreciate how radical the idea of experiential learning and reflection were when they were first proposed. Alexander Neill (1968) and Carl Rogers (1983) have been included in Figure 11.2 as influential thinkers because of their radical approach to education at the time. Both Rogers in the USA and Neill in the UK developed and applied Dewey's ideas to the education of children, advocating learning through discovery. Both held the belief that children learn best when they can see the relevance of what they are being asked to do; learning needed to be significant and meaningful for children. Again, it is necessary to emphasise how radical such an approach was. At a time when **learning by rote** was the general educational approach, any move to put children at the centre of their learning in order to make it meaningful was revolutionary. Both Neill and Rogers were arguing against the accepted approach of the time. Neill was the headmaster of Summerhill School in Suffolk, England, and believed that the school should be made to fit the child and not the other way around. This school still exists and has the ethos that lessons are optional; there is no pressure to conform to adult ideas of 'growing up'. There are, however, expectations of a standard of behaviour. At Summerhill, the importance of expressing emotions and learning through feelings is clearly recognised.

The approach of giving individuals freedom to learn and moving away from learning by rote was later adopted within adult learning, and then further developed and applied to the education of professionals. Looking back from our current position of undertaking reflection as a requirement to maintain nursing registration (NMC, 2016), the radical heritage of reflection, a process in which we freely focus upon aspects of learning we decide are necessary, now seems implausible.

Reflection is a process that we all, to some extent, engage in naturally. It is human nature to ponder experience, asking questions such as 'What did I do well?' and 'Why did I, or others, respond like that?'. The challenge we face when trying to answer such questions is that definitive responses may not exist. Thus, we have to accept that the thinking and learning resulting from reflection, is based on speculation.

ACTIVITY 11.2

- Do you think there could be any dangers in using information based upon speculation?
- Provide a rationale for your answer.

Check the activity answers at the end of the chapter to see if our thoughts are similar.

We discussed speculation in Chapter 3 in consideration of its role in critical thinking. In the critical thinking we undertake in reflection, we need to apply informed speculation. We are not just thinking randomly, but making deliberate links to relevant information. Speculation is a good way to be creative in our thinking, but we must ensure that we don't make links between ideas that are actually without a proven relationship to each other. Figure 11.3 identifies examples of how linking ideas without a proven relationship can lead to invalid assumptions.

Swans are white.

Twinkle is white, so she is a swan.

Nurses wear uniforms.

Sarah wears a uniform, so she is a nurse.

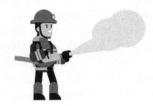

Frogs have 4 legs.

Fifi has 4 legs so she is a frog.

Figure 11.3   Invalid assumptions

FEELINGS AND EMOTIONS

Earlier in the chapter we mentioned that at Summerhill School the importance of expressing emotions and learning through feelings was clearly recognised. This approach translates directly into how we apply reflective practice. According to Schön (1987, p. 200), expert nurse practitioners not only know how to apply their theoretical knowledge, but they are able to demonstrate competencies such as 'intuition', 'talent' and 'wisdom' in challenging situations. They have been able to reach a state of professional artistry based on using reflective practice to tap into their feelings and emotions in order to learn from experience. Emotions and feelings are seen as important in reflection and are actively considered. Emotions not only influence the way we think, but also our beliefs, values and attitudes. The emotional perspective is clearly valued in experiential learning. This is in direct contrast to traditional academic thinking where, when we write about ideas, we are required to do so from an objective, unbiased perspective. In a traditional academic approach, emotion is viewed as limiting the development of knowledge.

Consideration of an experiential learning approach in contrast to a traditional academic approach highlights further issues. As we discussed in Chapter 9, evidence-based practice has been accused of valuing scientific research evidence more highly than evidence gained from reflection – in other words, nursing expertise. While we may view these two elements to be so deeply intertwined that they form two parts of one whole, this view is not unanimously accepted, as shown in Figure 11.4.

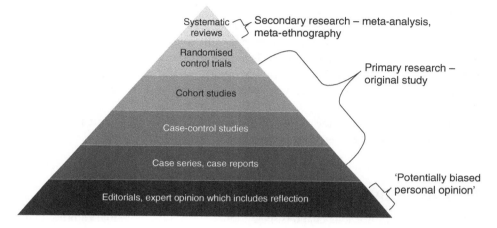

Figure 11.4   The position of reflection in the hierarchy of evidence

Within the hierarchy of evidence, reflection is viewed as potentially biased personal opinion and ranked within the category of least value. So, although reflection has been clearly adopted in nursing and identified as being fundamental in good practice (NMC, 2016), its value is yet to be fully recognised within **academia**. For some, reflection still remains too radical a concept to fully recognise.

While progress has been made in implementing Schön's approach and valuing more than pure knowledge alone, reflection could be seen as occupying the position of 'another technical tool' (Rolfe, 2002, p. 21). It is nearly 20 years since Rolfe described reflection as 'another technical tool' and the state remains unchanged. Knowledge generated by practitioners reflecting on their own experiences is still not viewed to be of equal value to knowledge derived from **empirical** research. As we have highlighted, there have been steps forward – for example, reflection becoming a mandatory requirement (NMC, 2016). However, this may itself perpetuate Rolfe's view. If nurses are applying reflection in a mechanistic manner because 'they have to' using 'another technical tool', the true potential of reflective practice still remains undiscovered.

FURTHER WORK TO BE DONE

Looking to the future and learning from the past, there are clear lessons. Undertaking reflective practice can be daunting and confusing. There remains the need for a guide, be that a lecturer, a textbook, an experienced colleague or a combination of all of these. The question is, 'What is the way forward?'. Future nurses need to be efficient information navigators, effective team members and compassionate care givers, while maintaining their well-being and avoiding burnout (Ross and Derouin, 2018). Reflection can assist in building these behaviours, enabling the development of thoughtful choices for future action, increasing self-awareness and understanding the importance of self-care. However, as Rolfe (2014, p. 1182) eloquently cautions:

> *true reflective practice is being squeezed out of our nursing and healthcare departments as a result of a very narrow and misguided concept of what academic research and scholarship should look like.*

While it is more than six years since Rolfe made this comment, it remains appropriate. Again, as outlined by Rolfe (2014), what is needed is for nursing academics and practitioners to assert a scholarship of practice in tandem with the existing theoretical and research-based scholarship. In this way, both the science and artistry of nursing can, rightly, be equally valued.

Reflective practice has come a long way from its radical beginnings, but as yet neither the journey nor its radical reach are complete.

IS IT ALL GOOD?

As we have said in previous chapters, being reflective has the potential to bring many benefits. You are able to learn from experience rather than just 'being on auto-pilot', which results in deep rather than surface learning. The differences between these two types of learning are highlighted in Figure 11.5.

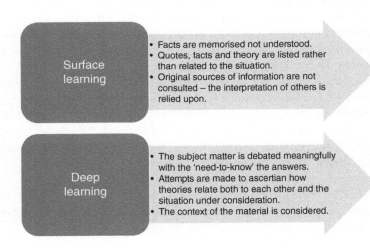

Figure 11.5   The differences between surface and deep learning

Source: Adapted from Biggs and Tang (2007)

The learning you gain from effective reflection is deep learning because you are focusing on an experience with the desire to make sense and meaning from it. Thus, when you engage with relevant theory in your reflection, this becomes meaningful and you have the desire to find answers to the questions you ask.

Reflective learning enables you to identify your strengths and areas where you need further development, plus your self-awareness is increased as you are assisted to become aware of your beliefs, attitudes and values. Becoming reflective in your approach to experience encourages self-directed learning, motivates you to seek feedback on your actions, and thus improves your personal and professional confidence and competence.

As Oscar asks at the start of the chapter, however, can it really all be positive? The key to making positive gains from reflection is in ensuring that it is effective. There are a number of potential limitations and challenges that may hamper your ability to reflect effectively (Boud and Walker, 1998), as identified in Table 11.1.

Table 11.1   Reflection: limitations and challenges

Limitations	Challenges
Reflection undertaken in a mechanical fashion ('going through the motions') so that the resulting reflective practice is ineffective.	Not understanding what reflection means and what the reflective process involves.
Getting 'stuck' in the reflective process and being uncertain how to proceed in order to further develop your thinking.	Not having the support needed to assist with the reflective process or implementing a plan of action resulting from the reflection.
Having to reflect rather than wanting to – for example, having to produce a reflection for an assignment without appreciating the benefit of it.	Finding the time and having the motivation to reflect.
Lack of honesty, which can be: • unconscious, where you don't perceive there is a need for improvement; • conscious, where you perceive there is a need for improvement, but decide not to address it.	Fear of being: • criticised because the focus of the reflection is on a lack of knowledge or skill; • seen as arrogant because the focus of the reflection is on being proficient.

Reflecting effectively is far from a simple process. To reflect, you need a wide range of pre-existing academic skills or the support from others to assist you to attain these skills. As Charlie said at the start of the chapter, undertaking a reflection can make your head hurt, because in order to attain a deep level of learning you need to actively engage with the material and think critically about it.

ACTIVITY 11.3

Review the information presented in Table 11.1.

*   Can you identify strategies you could apply in order to overcome each of the limitations or challenges?

Check the activity answers at the end of the chapter to see if our thoughts are similar.

Reflecting on experience may be negatively influenced by a lack of objectivity and an inability to perceive areas of weakness or attitudes, decisions and values that are not positive. Further to this, we reflect by reconstructing an experience, rather than having an accurate record of the situation. Our reconstructions can encourage us to focus on negative emotions and thus adversely impact our well-being. However, the consideration of our feelings and emotions within a reflection is fundamental to the process. This alone presents a challenge because the ability to consider personal emotions from an objective perspective is a highly advanced academic skill. It is possible, however, with support and guidance, to acknowledge the potential negative consequences and have the motivation to master the difficulties so that reflection can become an excellent approach to learning about ourselves and gain meaning from experience.

CONCLUSION

When we reflect, we are creating our own reality by making sense of experience – an approach that is not only a continuous process, but also echoes a number of spiritual teachings.

In essence, reflective practice is a development of the theory of learning from experience. The application of this approach facilitates a process of personal and professional learning which constantly alters our views.

The history of reflective practice can be traced as far back as the work of Socrates, the Greek philosopher, and his 'Socratic questioning'. In later times, the work of Dewey (1933) and Schön (1983, 1987) was fundamental to the development of reflective practice as we know it. The work of Schön in particular was central to the realisation that professionals required more than pure theory alone in order to be able to function proficiently. At a time when reflective practice is a mandatory aspect of revalidation for every nurse registered in the UK and other countries, learning that reflection has a radical heritage may well be unexpected. Reflective practice has come a long way from its origins of being a ground-breaking new approach, developed from a method of learning that was contrary to the accepted norm. However, there is danger in reflective practice being a mandatory aspect of revalidation, but also in the many assessments required to complete nursing programmes. Such an approach brings the potential that a method of learning with enlightening possibilities could be undertaken in a mechanistic fashion, thus devaluing its worth.

The academic skill to be able to learn objectively from feelings and emotions required in reflective practice is one that takes time and practice to master. Evidence from effective reflection can, however, bring value not only to individual nursing practice and patient care, but to academia also. The acceptance of the true value of knowledge based on reflection within academia remains an ongoing challenge. There is still work to do.

GOING FURTHER

Dewey, J. (1933) *How We Think*. Boston, MA: DC Heath & Co. Dewey's seminal text, from which reflection as we know it today developed.

Ixer, G. (1999) There's no such thing as reflection. *British Journal of Social Work*, 29: 513-27. An interesting article which, although it is more than ten years old, still provides a relevant overview of the problem with reflective practice.

The danger of wild speculation. Go to: www.youtube.com/watch?v=H9PY_3E3h2c. We have considered the importance of ensuring within reflections that we link our ideas carefully and ensure that there is an accurate relationship. This classic Monty Python clip identifies exactly where we end up when we apply faulty reasoning.

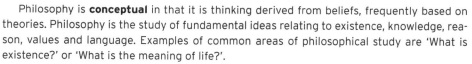

ANSWERS TO ACTIVITIES

Activity 11.1

There is a difference between the definition of theory and philosophy, which it is useful to appreciate.

Philosophy is **conceptual** in that it is thinking derived from beliefs, frequently based on theories. Philosophy is the study of fundamental ideas relating to existence, knowledge, reason, values and language. Examples of common areas of philosophical study are 'What is existence?' or 'What is the meaning of life?'.

Theory is a practical explanation of how something works. Theories are interpretations that make an idea clearer and are based on evidence rather than belief. Examples of well-known theory are the theory of evolution or the theory of gravity.

Activity 11.2

In Chapter 3 we considered the role of speculation in critical thinking. When we speculate, we are presenting ideas based on the best knowledge we have. In reflections, speculating is important because it enables you to identify both what might be happening and what could be possible. Thus, speculation can assist to explain problems, help you to find solutions for them and identify strategies to explore other future possibilities.

There is, however, danger if your speculation is not informed. We need to ensure that the ideas we present in our speculation are actually relevant and based on the best knowledge we have, so our speculation is informed and not wild guessing.

Activity 11.3

It can be difficult to overcome all the limitations and challenges we identified. There are, however, a number of strategies that might be helpful, as identified in Table 11.2, that you could implement as well as those you suggested.

(Continued)

Table 11.2   Reflection: strategies to assist you to overcome limitations and challenges

Limitations	Challenges
Reflection undertaken in a mechanical fashion ('going through the motions') so that the resulting reflective practice is ineffective.	Not understanding what reflection means and what the reflective process involves.
Strategy	*Strategy*
It sounds as if there is little motivation to reflect and a lack of understanding of the process. In this situation it would be helpful to gain a greater understanding of the process of reflection and focus on the potential personal and professional benefit that reflection brings.	*Again, it seems as if there is a need for a greater understanding of reflection in general and more specifically an increase in the knowledge of how to apply the chosen model.*
Getting 'stuck' in the reflective process and being uncertain how to proceed in order to further develop your thinking.	Not having the support needed to assist with the reflective process or implementing a plan of action resulting from the reflection.
Strategy	*Strategy*
It could be of great benefit to find another individual who you trust and has a good understanding of reflection to help. You could either ask them to read your reflection or talk it through with them, identifying where you felt 'stuck' and asking for their advice as to how you could move forwards.	*This is actually a common challenge that novice reflectors face. Reflection is frequently discussed as an individual undertaking, but when you are starting to develop your reflective skills in particular, it is good to find another, more experienced person, who you trust and is willing to support you. With their support. you will be able to develop your reflections and work on the resulting plan of action.*
Having to reflect rather than wanting to, for example, have to produce a reflection for an assignment without appreciating the benefit of this.	Finding the time and having the motivation to reflect.
Strategy	*Strategy*
You need to find a way of reflecting that you think does at least offer you some benefits. We have considered a range of models in this textbook, and there are many more available. It might also be helpful to reflect with another person, or even a group of people. This may enable you to feel that you are gaining something from the process rather than just going through the motions.	*We have all experienced this challenge – time and motivation can be in short supply as you try to combine a busy work life, home life and study.*
	Motivation can be gained from thinking about the benefit of reflecting and choosing an experience to reflect on what you are passionate about.
	Making time to reflect is possible if you make use of every opportunity. Think carefully through your day to discover time that can be used for reflective thinking – for example, when you are walking the dog, doing the washing up, waiting for the children while they are at football. Make sure that you always have a notebook with you to be able to record your thinking or use the voice memo function on your phone and speak your thoughts.

Limitations	Challenges
Lack of honesty, which can be:	Fear of being:

Lack of honesty, which can be:

- unconscious, where you don't perceive there is a need for improvement;
- conscious, where you perceive there is a need for improvement, but decide not to address it.

Fear of being:

- criticised because the focus of the reflection is on a lack of knowledge or skill;
- seen as arrogant because the focus of the reflection is on being proficient.

Strategy

You can help yourself to become aware of areas for improvement you haven't previously been able to perceive by sharing your reflections with another person or persons who are able to assist you to identify these areas. It would be important that you trusted the other person or persons and felt able to act on the suggestions they made.

If you purposefully decide not to acknowledge a need for improvement, it is important to be honest with yourself as to why this is. It may be that you wish to develop other areas first, which is a sensible strategy.

If you realise that you are not addressing issues which are negatively influencing your practice, remember that at all times you need to uphold The Code (NMC, 2018). If you are aware of a learning need, to abide by the Code you must address it. You are not alone when working on your professional development, so discuss your concern with a trusted colleague, supervisor or lecturer.

Strategy

To reflect effectively, we need to be willing to share our areas of both weakness and strength. It can be scary to do this, either because you feel that you should know more than you do, or because you don't want others to think that you 'know everything'. Remember, however, that it is your choice what you decide to share. While you may undertake reflection as an assessment, you choose the experience you reflect on.

Reflection is an effective way to consider experiences that you find personally emotive, but you choose who you share this with. Such a reflection would be something to share with those you trust most, but possibly not something to focus on for other purposes.

GLOSSARY

academia The environment or community concerned with the pursuit of research, education and scholarship.

concept Idea or thought.

conceptual Based on ideas or thoughts.

empirical Based on observation and/or evidence.

facilitates Makes an action or a process easier.

learning by rote Memorising facts by repetition. The idea is that you will be able to quickly recall the meaning of the material the more that you repeat it.

REFERENCES

Biggs, J.B. and Tang, C. (2007) *Teaching for Quality Learning at University* (3rd edn). Maidenhead: Open University Press.

Boud, D. and Walker, D. (1998) Promoting reflection in professional courses: the challenge of context. *Studies in Higher Education*, 23(2): 191–206.

Dewey, J. (1933) *How We Think*. Boston, MA: Heath & Co.

Gibbs, G. (1988) *Learning by Doing: A Guide to Teaching and Learning Methods*. Further Education Unit, Oxford Polytechnic, Oxford.

Johns, C. (2017) *Becoming a Reflective Practitioner*. Oxford: Wiley-Blackwell.

Kant, I. (1889) (trans. T.K. Abbott) *Critique of Practical Reason and Other Works and the Theory of Ethics*. London: Longman.

Kolb, D.A. (1984) *Experiential Learning: Experience as the Source of Learning and Development*. Englewood Cliffs, NJ: Prentice-Hall.

Neill, A.S. (1968) *Summerhill*. Harmondsworth: Penguin.

Nursing and Midwifery Council (NMC) (2016) Revalidation/What you need to do. Written reflective accounts. Available at: http://revalidation.nmc.org.uk/what-you-need-to-do/written-reflective-accounts/ (accessed 19 August 2020).

Rogers, C. (1983) *Freedom to Learn for the 80's*. Columbus, OH: Charles E. Merrill Publishing Co.

Rolfe, G. (2002) Reflective practice: where now? *Nurse Education in Practice*, 2: 21–9.

Rolfe, G. (2014) Rethinking reflective education: what would Dewey have done? *Nurse Education Today*, 34: 1179–83.

Ross, E. and Derouin, A. (2018) Fostering reflective future healthcare professionals. *Medical Science Educator*, 28: 9–10.

Schön, D.A. (1983) *The Reflective Practitioner: How Professionals Think in Action*. London: Maurice Temple Smith.

Schön, D.A. (1987) *Educating the Reflective Practitioner*. San Francisco, CA: Jossey Bass.

INDEX

Numbers in **bold** denote glossary enties